# Best Practices in Medical Teaching

# Best Practices in Medical Teaching

Stephen M. Stahl

and

Richard L. Davis

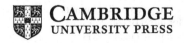

# CAMBRIDGE
## UNIVERSITY PRESS

University Printing House, Cambridge CB2 8BS, United Kingdom

One Liberty Plaza, 20th Floor, New York, NY 10006, USA

477 Williamstown Road, Port Melbourne, VIC 3207, Australia

314-321, 3rd Floor, Plot 3, Splendor Forum, Jasola District Centre, New Delhi - 110025, India

79 Anson Road, #06-04/06, Singapore 079906

Cambridge University Press is part of the University of Cambridge.

It furthers the University's mission by disseminating knowledge in the pursuit of
education, learning and research at the highest international levels of excellence.

www.cambridge.org
Information on this title: www.cambridge.org/9780521151764

© Arbor Scientia 2011

First published 2011
Reprinted 2017

*A catalogue record for this publication is available from the British Library*

*Library of Congress Cataloging in Publication data*
Stahl, S. M.
Best practices in medical teaching / Stephen M. Stahl and Richard L. Davis.
    p. ; cm.
Includes bibliographical references and index.
ISBN 978-0-521-15176-4 (pbk.)
1. Medical education.   2. Teaching.   I. Davis, Richard L., 1954–   II. Title.
[DNLM: 1. Education, Medical – methods.   2. Multimedia.   3. Teaching – methods. W 18]
R735.S73   2011
610.71–dc22

2011010560

ISBN 978-0-521-15176-4 Paperback

........................................................................................................

# Contents

# Preface

This book was conceived and developed to be a change agent for medical educators. We hope that the principles, concepts and illustrations contained within will raise the effectiveness of those who teach. One might consider the contents of this book to be the "rest of the story" concerning current medical education practices. That is, the tools presented in this book are intended to be the communication complement to the traditional subject matter content of medical education. The premise of this book is that combining the science of communication with the communication of science creates an incrementally more valuable exchange for both the instructor and the learner.

Hopefully there will be something in this book for everyone, from novice instructors to the most experienced mentors. Novice medical educators may discover many new principles about how to assist others to learn. In fact, this book is organized with the first section examining how to apply the principles of adult learning to the design of effective educational presentations. The second section focuses on gaining an understanding of the many and various aspects of the different learners represented in any medical audience. This is followed in the third section by information on the instructor's performance and the impact it can have on effectiveness. The last area discussed is how to measure and evaluate educational programs to see if they have reached their desired outcomes. Each chapter is followed by a knowledge check and an assessment section. Novices will find it useful to work through the book from beginning to end, checking their progress along the way to make sure that key concepts are understood.

Seasoned medical educators may find thought-provoking principles that they will immediately recognize as scientific explanations for concepts they have instinctively used in their own teaching. Veteran instructors may find that a more expedient use of the book would be to peruse the table of contents of each chapter to find specific areas of interest or challenge to examine. Another approach might be to go the Progress Check and Assessment at the end of each chapter to help identify the area of greatest value for time spent.

Whether novice or experienced, you will find that this book will lead you to become an increasingly more effective educator. In so doing, you will better serve not only those you instruct but ultimately the many patients that your audience members will treat.

Best wishes as you endeavor to enhance your capabilities and educational performance and thank you for serving the medical field through your instructional efforts.

Stephen M. Stahl, MD, PhD
Founder,
Neuroscience Education Institute

Richard L. Davis
President
Arbor Scientia

# About the authors

**Dr. Stephen M. Stahl** has held faculty positions at Stanford University, the University of California at Los Angeles, the Institute of Psychiatry London, the Institute of Neurology London, and, currently, at the University of California at San Diego. Recently, Dr. Stahl was elected an Honorary Visiting Senior Fellow in the Department of Psychiatry and a Visiting Fellow at Clare Hall at the University of Cambridge in the UK. Dr. Stahl was also Executive Director of Clinical Neurosciences at the Merck Neuroscience Research Center in the UK for several years. Dr. Stahl's major interests are dedicated to producing and disseminating educational information about diseases and their treatments in psychiatry and neurology, with a special emphasis on multimedia, the internet, and teaching how to teach.

Dr. Stahl has conducted numerous research projects during his career awarded by the National Institute of Mental Health, by the Veterans Administration and by the pharmaceutical industry. Author of over 425 articles and chapters, and more than 1500 scientific presentations and abstracts, Dr. Stahl is an internationally recognized clinician, researcher, and teacher in psychiatry with subspecialty expertise in psychopharmacology. Dr. Stahl has edited five books and written 25 others, of which hundreds of thousands have been sold, including the best-selling textbook *Stahl's Essential Psychopharmacology*, now in its third edition, and the best-selling clinical manual *Stahl's Essential Psychopharmacology Prescriber's Guide*, now in its fourth edition, winner of the British Medical Association's Pharmacology Book of the Year award.

Lectures, courses, and preceptorships based upon his textbooks have taken him to dozens of countries on six continents to speak to tens of thousands of physicians, mental health professionals, and students at all levels. His lectures and scientific presentations have been distributed as millions of CD-ROMs, internet educational programs, videotapes, audiotapes, and programmed home-study texts for continuing medical education to hundreds of thousands of professionals in many different languages. His courses and award-winning multimedia teaching materials are used by psychopharmacology teachers and students throughout the world. Dr. Stahl also writes didactic features for mental health professionals in numerous journals.

His educational research programs are monitoring changes in diagnosing and prescribing behaviors as outcomes from various educational interventions for programs organized by the Neuroscience Education Institute, an award-winning ACCME educational provider, accredited with commendation, which he chairs. He also has an active clinical practice specializing in psychopharmacologic treatment of resistant cases.

He has been named recipient of the International College of Neuropsychopharmacology (CINP) Lundbeck Foundation Award in Education for his contributions to postgraduate education in psychiatry and neurology, and also the winner of the A. E. Bennett Award of the Society of Biological Psychiatry, the American Psychiatric Association/San Diego Psychiatric Society Education Award, and has been cited as both one of "America's Top Psychiatrists" and one of the "Best Doctors in America."

**Richard L. Davis** is president of Arbor Scientia, a global medical communications company headquartered in Carlsbad, California, and winner of the Carlsbad Chamber of Commerce's Business of the Year award.

His experience with the pharmaceutical industry spans over 15 years. Mr. Davis has developed a number of innovative education programs at Arbor Scientia and highly sought-after programs on principles of adult education, the role of personality profiles in audience psychology and speaker effectiveness, and teaching how to teach. He is a member of the American Society of Training and Development.

Lectures, courses, and coaching sessions based upon his work and publications have taken him to dozens of countries on five continents to speak to thousands of physicians and medical professionals. Mr. Davis has been a featured speaker on the topic of instructional design at the CINP Biennial meeting, and is also a highly sought-after executive coach, providing dozens of speakers and top executives and medical professionals in multiple therapeutic areas with personal executive coaching including consultations on presentation skills.

His educational programs have been cited by the San Diego Branch of the American Psychiatric Association for excellence in medical education and by the CINP (International College of Neuropsychopharmacology) for postgraduate education in neurology and psychiatry.

# Foreword

Maestro Stahl has done it again. Instead of educating us on cutting-edge theory and pragmatics of neuropsychopharmacology, he is taking it one step further, teaching us how to better educate others. The target audience for this timely, concise, yet comprehensive pearl is medical educators, but the lessons he and Richard Davis illustrate are applicable to a much broader audience. Stephen Stahl is widely regarded as one of the best, most effective and most influential teachers of contemporary psychopharmacology. On these pages, like a master pitching coach, he breaks down the essential mechanics, step by step, of effective pedagogy and delivery. Even novices, as well as the already established teachers, can assimilate the message, apply the material and improve their game.

He walks the walk and talks the talk. One of the most important aspects of this book is that it is written in precisely the way Stahl and Davis agree presentations should be made. There is an initial "grabber" set in the Preface, telling the reader why it's so important to attend to what he or she is about to read. Then there's a middle section, with lots of repetition and self-assessment tools to make sure the reader understands the material and plans to use it. Finally, there are ample summaries, posttests, and evaluations. Each lesson is well illustrated with the kind of graphics that clarify and amplify the written word and the lessons are broken down in manageable bits that don't overwhelm the reader.

One of the most memorable aspects of the book is the homage paid to other master educators and theorists, with frequent insets providing pictures, brief biographies, and key contributions of several icons in adult education theory. There are also pithy, often humorous quotes, including several from one of my personal favorites, Yogi Berra, to illuminate the message.

In short, the book not only describes how to become a powerful public speaker but also provides a living example of "best practices of medical education."

*But where were you when I needed you most?* My only regret is that I have been teaching for more than 30 years without this guidebook. I have no doubt I could have been a more effective instructor, in both small and large group settings, if something like this book had been available earlier in my career. It is a first of its kind! As a residency training director, I will make sure my trainees don't have the same regret. I plan to institute a course on "effective teaching," using this book as the primary source, to help residents learn valuable lessons for the work they do teaching students, other residents, staff and, to some extent, even their patients. This is a text every training director and medical educator should own.

Sidney Zisook, MD, Professor of Psychiatry
Director, Residency Training
University of California San Diego

# Acknowledgments

To Cindy, Jennifer and Victoria for their tireless support; to all medical educators for their contributions large and small, seen and unseen; and to my coauthor for opening my eyes to the science of communication and to the relentless pursuit of excellence in teaching. (Stephen M. Stahl)

This book is dedicated to my wife, Nathalie, who has been my partner, provoker and biggest supporter for 32 years; to my daughters, Nathalie and Rica, who motivate me in the way they conquer their challenges; and to my coauthor whose commitment to serving the field of medicine is inspirational and whose productivity is astonishing. Steve, thanks for another exciting outcome of our 14 year collaboration. (Richard L. Davis)

We would like to thank a group of individuals who played an important part in the completion of this book: Dana Wise, Matt Maneen, Dennis Kim and Nicole Gellings-Lowe, whose assistance in completing the book is much appreciated; Daniel Lara Rios for all of his great work on the graphics; Sharon Odegaard and Christa Tiernan for all their editing efforts; and Jennifer Stahl and Heather Dailey, whose tireless and relentless project management efforts kept us all on task and brought things to completion.

# Introduction

Medical education is a lifelong process. There is too much information and not enough time. Often, the response to this continuous explosion of knowledge is to try to shoehorn the maximum amount of content into every minute of every presentation and into every corner of every figure and every page. This attention to subject matter content is understandable but can often be self-defeating. It can even lead to inadvertent "audience abuse." That is, more content can actually lead to less learning if the content is made available but is not well designed. The point is not to present information but to get learners to remember and use it.

This book will consider whether the focus of medical education should be the medical content, the medical educator who does the presenting, or the learner. The perspective here is that the focus of medical education should be the learner and that the content should be structured and executed in a manner that facilitates learning instead of inhibiting it. However, the current system of medical education is often deficient in that it provides its instructors with only some of the skill set necessary to deliver the medical education needed. That is, plenty of attention is given to "what is said," but often little consideration is given to "how it is said." Evolving principles from communications science now inform us that such an approach can needlessly compromise the potential benefit of any educational effort for those it is intended to inform.

What a paradox that a field whose goal is to communicate science to its practitioners would not apply communication science in doing it. It is also illogical to expect those tasked with delivering the education to do so effectively with little to no exposure to the science that would empower them to do it in the most effective manner. A misplaced focus on content to the exclusion of the learner often lies at the heart of ineffective medical education, so changing that focus to the learner can bring about much-needed improvement in medical education from the learner's perspective.

This book was thus developed to be a tool for all those who undertake the task of helping other clinicians hone their skills through medical education. Specifically, we discuss how to apply the principles of communication science and propose some tips for how an instructor can develop best practices in medical education. This book supplies scientific tools and knowledge that can:

- Elevate and differentiate an instructor's skills
- Assist in the effective transfer of knowledge and skills from an instructor to a learner
- Increase the influence and impact of an instructor's presentation
- Create greater demand for an instructor and elevate the direct and perceived value of the education the instructor delivers

The excitement that comes from new levels of understanding and the increased proficiency associated with putting that understanding to work are benefits that both the medical instructor and the audience will share. Medical educators in fact are increasingly being made accountable for demonstrating that these new levels of understanding have occurred and that they have been put to work in the learner's medical practice. Documentation of the outcomes of medical education is the new standard that is evolving in this field, and it serves to make educators accountable for the effectiveness of their programs. Accountability for the results of a medical education program, however, does not rest solely on the shoulders of the instructor conveying the content but also on the shoulders of those who develop, design, and regulate the content to be covered.

Many of those with whom we have worked in live programs have shared with us that the communication principles to which they were introduced have influenced not only the effectiveness of their presentations but also their professional satisfaction from teaching others. We have distilled these principles in this book, and it is our goal to help as many as possible have a similar experience.

# Applying the principles of adult education to the designing of medical presentations

## Chapter overview

Chapter 1 introduces several critical learning principles that can be applied when designing a medical presentation and that have the potential of increasing the impact of individual slides, entire slide decks, and even entire educational events (see Stahl and Davis, 2009a).

The first section discusses storyboarding, with emphasis on **previews and reviews**. A preview facilitates learner achievement by acting as a roadmap to alert audiences about important topics to come. Repeated reviews help ensure that messages are clearly delivered by providing a second chance for learning, by helping learners consolidate information, and by clarifying outstanding issues.

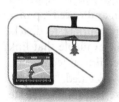

Between previews and reviews, delivering information in **small multiples** gives learners manageable packets of data and helps them to see differences as well as similarities between conditions. The second section discusses how to organize the words of text and especially images as a sequence of small multiples to enhance impact.

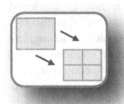

The majority of audience members prefer visual components in their learning materials, so adding relevant images and figures can increase learning impact. The section on **visual additions** discusses how to provide visual cues without distractions or data decorations.

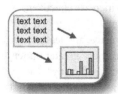

**Principles of multimedia learning** can help guide instructional design to best utilize these technologies. To increase the impact of presentations, information can be presented in both auditory and visual channels in ways that eliminate

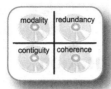

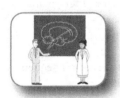

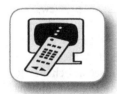

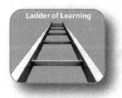

interference from the textual channel, present related information in close spatial and temporal proximity, and eliminate extraneous information.

**Educational design principles** suggest advantages to delivering information in order to gain and control attention, describe expected outcomes, and refer to previous learning – all of which would ideally be addressed before new information is presented. Then, after new information is presented, impact is heightened by medical educators supplying guidance for learning, appraising performance, giving feedback, and providing for the transfer of knowledge into clinical practice.

The classical **conditions of learning** are involving learners and getting them to invest in their own learning by challenging their knowledge, yet providing support within a structured format, generating feedback, and supplying opportunities for practical application. These facilitation techniques help learners to integrate their current knowledge with new information.

Providing feedback to learners helps them assess their own learning and is an extremely important milestone in adult education. An **audience response keypad system** can provide appropriate feedback. Small, portable systems are now available that link to PowerPoint and do not require a technician. When properly designed and executed, audience response questions can increase learning, generate interactivity, and measure progress.

Once a high-quality presentation is developed, working with a second medical instructor, as discussed in the section on **team and tandem teaching**, can make an educational event more engaging for the audience and help accommodate attention spans.

Medical educators may wish to move away occasionally from traditional lecture presentations to even **higher-impact learning formats**, which can be incorporated into an educational event to increase effectiveness. Research into instructional design has suggested that educational formats that are more active and less passive for the learners may result in the learners' greater understanding, longer retention, and increased enjoyment.

One tactic for creating a learning format with demonstrated superior efficacy in medical

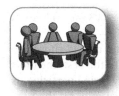

education is to **design and facilitate workshops or discussion groups**. Workshops involve putting content into the hands of the learners and asking them to examine and contribute to the material. When properly managed by an effective facilitator, workshops can create a more effective learning environment than traditional lectures or presentations. In addition, they can elevate the audience's perception of both the instructor's competence and the presentation's value.

A **progress check** section is included to allow review and application of the key principles of adult education that are explored in Chapter 1.

# Introduction

## Rationale and benefits

### It's all in the setup

To paraphrase the baseball great and folk philosopher Yogi Berra, teaching is 90% preparation; the other 50% is execution. This chapter will emphasize preparation – namely, those scientific principles that can guide the designing of medical presentations. Later chapters will deal more directly with the execution of medical presentations.

Essentially all medical educators communicate scientific information and data because they are recognized content matter experts. However, many medical educators are not necessarily experts in the scientific principles of adult learning because in medicine, most experts are not taught how to teach per se.

"See one, do one, teach one" is the basic tenet. "Understand first, then as an expert, one can be understood as a teacher" is the classical notion in medical education. Many effective medical educators simply follow personal instincts and thus design educational programs intuitively while adapting the educational style and principles of mentors who were influential in their own careers.

This approach works for many, especially those with natural talents and charisma. However, there exist numerous scientific principles based upon data from educational research studies that, if applied, can raise the effectiveness of any teacher. This chapter is about those principles. In other words, here we discuss how to communicate the science by using the science of communication.

### What is the focus?

Preparation begins with answering this question. The explosion of information in medicine and the sheer volume of information cause the focus of most medical education programs to be **content**. Some estimates are that every year, trillions of new statistical graphics are printed (Tufte, 1983).

Content often flows from carefully constructed curricula and is chosen to foster the development of experts by exposing participants to the best, the most up-to-date, and the most important content. This is done by giving participants the greatest breadth and depth of content exposure, limited only by the time available.

If it's all about the content, then the more content, the better. However, poorly designed graphics often distort the data, leaving the wrong impression. Also, cramming too much content into slides and too many words into a rapid-fire lecture can cause audience frustration due to the participants' inability to process or retain the vast volume of information presented.

One creative solution to the problem of too much information was witnessed by one of the authors recently. He arrived at a large hall, expecting to give a guest lecture in basic pharmacology to a class of 150 medical students. But only a dozen students were in the audience. One prominent audience member sat in the middle of the front row with an MP3 recorder and a horde of handouts. When questioned, the student said that the class had determined that the most important aspect of the lectures were the handouts because these formed the basis of exam questions. Students believed that lectures were generally given too fast and in too disorganized a fashion for effective learning. Thus, they had determined that the option of being able to play back some lectures at a later time, after previewing the relevant handouts, and with the ability to replay important points at one's own learning pace, was the best way to learn the material. So they all took turns recording lectures and procuring handouts, allowing them the freedom of spending the lecture time more productively studying by themselves.

This may be an extreme example, but it could cause a medical educator to wonder whether less content is, in fact, actually more in terms of learning. Indeed, principles of adult learning underscore that this is true, as will be discussed in subsequent chapters.

The question is, then: If content should not be the focus, what should be?

**Presenter focus.** One solution is to have a "presenter focus" to education, letting the expert choose the topic and the manner of presentation. Content matter experts in medical topics are rare, busy, and highly sought after. This solution is sometimes the only way to cajole these experts into giving a presentation. In academic medicine, education is often neither respected nor richly rewarded. Some say that in medicine, research flies first class, clinical care and administration fly coach, and education is often just cargo. Perhaps this is also the basis of the adage: "Those who can, do; those who can't, teach."

A presenter focus to medical education can work well if there are enough experts with natural teaching skills available, but it can also yield some off-beat presentations. The expert may enjoy the ease of preparation but the curriculum and the learners may not be well served.

Also, such presenter-focused experts may assume that others learn in the same way they do, so they will teach the same way they learn. In later chapters, this book will cover the flaws in this rationale, showing that, in a typical audience, many have learning styles that differ from those of the presenter.

**Participant or learner focus.** If the purpose of medical education is not only exposure to content but also learning and using the content, then a "participant focus" or a "learner focus" could be the best option. This means there is more work to be done after the content has been selected. The presenter will also have the task of organizing the content to maximize the number of participants in the audience who will learn the material, retain it, and apply it.

Ironically, successful presentations designed with a participant focus are likely to be even more content-focused and presenter-focused than presentations designed from only one of those perspectives. What good is exposure to content if it is not remembered? What is the value of a presenter who designs lectures that are easy and interesting for the lecturer but fails to convince a participant to use the information? How successful is a presenter who is unable to assist a participant to develop a new skill or to change and upgrade clinical practice behaviors? In the participant-focused presentation, all three aspects can come together for greatest effectiveness.

To create a participant-focused presentation, a presenter can apply the general principles of adult learning to the overall design of presentations. This chapter introduces these principles and also suggests specific tweaks to slides, such as visual optimizations, that can enhance learning. Tips are given as well for using an audience response keypad system to document learning. A brief discussion of other education tactics such as converting lectures into workshops or team teaching is also included (see Stahl and Davis, 2009a).

## Section 1

### Storyboarding a medical presentation as a three-act play using previews and reviews

Lectures can be arranged as a dull recitation of facts or as a story that makes the facts come alive. Generally speaking, a participant is less interested in hearing the facts that an instructor has to present than in hearing a story the instructor has to tell. Organizing content into a "three-act play" can make a presentation memorable and its lessons practical. Some experts explain the three parts as: "Say what you're gonna say; say it; then say what you said." More specifically, the previews are the first part, the presentation itself is the second part, and the reviews are the third part of this structure.

Adding previews and reviews is one of the easiest ways to enhance the impact of a presentation. This can be done simply by following the old saw: "Begin with the end in mind." This involves previewing what the outcome of the presentation should be, then giving the lecture, and finally, emphasizing the key points and expected outcomes from the presentation with reviews.

### Previews

The standard format for the first "act" of a presentation is to list the objectives of the presentation. However, it is also possible to incorporate much more powerful previews or "hooks" that can propel the participant headfirst and with eagerness into the content that is about to follow.

When given previews, learners may perceive a medical instructor more positively because they see evidence of preparation (Chilcoat, 1989). The simplest place to start is to insert an outline slide at the beginning of the presentation. Then, have the outline recur at appropriate points throughout the deck to remind the audience of the topics ahead as well as those already discussed. The outline slide serves as a route map at the start and as a signpost at key intervals along the learning path.

Previews can also include a clinical anecdote, especially one from the presenter's own experience, that shows why the material is important or relevant.

Another option is to hook the audience in three steps: issue, action, and benefit. That is, state what the **issue** will be in the upcoming content, explain what **action** the participants should take, and finally, convince them to take this action by clearly showing the **benefits**.

This approach of preparing an intriguing first act with previews can prime the audience for the second and main act of the storyboard, namely, the content itself.

### Reviews

Reviews provide a second opportunity for learning. They allow an opportunity to clarify material for those who did not completely understand, to link cumulative presentation elements, and to help the audience members consolidate what they have learned (Chilcoat, 1989). Insertion of a summary or conclusion slide at the end of each section is the simplest way to address this tactic. A more elegant way is to remind the audience of the issues that were discussed, the actions that they should take, and why, by emphasizing the benefits to them of these actions.

### Section summary: storyboarding a medical presentation as a three-act play using previews and reviews

Previews facilitate learner achievement and may help learners view a medical instructor more positively; reviews also help consolidate audience learning and ensure that messages have been clearly delivered and received (see Stahl and Davis, 2009b).

## Section 2

### Organizing content as small multiples

The main part of the presentation, coming after it has been set up with a preview and a hook, is the body of the presentation itself. This content portion is the second and longest act of the three-act play.

**BIOBOX 1-1**

**Edward R. Tufte**

- Born 1942
- BA and MS in statistics from Stanford University
- PhD in political science from Yale University
- Professor of Political Economy and Data Analysis at Princeton University
- Currently Professor Emeritus of Statistics, Information Design, and Political Economy at Yale University
- Author of several books on information design and the visual presentation of data
- Called the "da Vinci of Data" by *The New York Times*

## Graphical excellence

As mentioned, if knowledge transfer rather than simple exposure to content is the goal, then it is important to optimize the visual presentation of data while avoiding overwhelming the audience with too much information all at once.

Edward Tufte is considered the champion of how best to represent data visually (BioBox 1-1). His 1983 book, *The Visual Display of Quantitative Information*, was named one of the 100 most important books published in the twentieth century.

Tufte is also credited with discovering why scientists did not foresee the Challenger space shuttle disaster, even though the data that predicted the failure of the famous o-rings were in plain sight of some of the smartest people in the world prior to the launch. They missed the predictable disaster because of the wrong graphical presentation of their data. Tufte discovered that when the data on o-ring damage were sequenced by date of launch, as they were prior to the fateful launch, this obscured the possible link between temperature and o-ring damage. When the evidence was placed in order by temperature, it was obvious that o-ring damage increased as temperature decreased. This was especially significant at temperatures below 65 degrees Fahrenheit, increasing damage progressively as temperatures declined to 52 degrees, the lowest temperature tested (Tufte, 1997). The scientists, however, missed this relationship and approved the launch at a temperature between 26 and 29 degrees, with catastrophic outcome. This is a powerful lesson in the value of graphical representation of data.

Some of the principles of graphical excellence proposed by Tufte are listed in Table 1-1. One of the central notions here is the emphasis on "data ink" (i.e., dots,

**TABLE 1-1:** Excellence in graphical displays

- ▸ Use complex ideas communicated with clarity, precision, and efficiency.
- ▸ Draw the viewer's attention to the sense and substance of the data.
- ▸ Show the data with a high proportion of data ink.
- ▸ Emphasize data ink (such as dots, lines, and labels; the nonerasable core of a graphic; and the non-redundant ink arranged in response to variation in the numbers represented).
- ▸ De-emphasize non-data ink (such as the title, the abscissa, the ordinate, and their labels).
- ▸ Change data ink as the data change.
- ▸ Induce the viewer to think about substance rather than methodology, graphic design, the technology of graphic production, or something else.
- ▸ Avoid distorting what the data have to say.
- ▸ Maximize data density and the size of the data matrix, within reason.
- ▸ Make large data sets coherent.
- ▸ Encourage the eye to compare different pieces of data.
- ▸ Reveal the data at several levels of detail, from a broad overview to the fine structure.
- ▸ Serve a reasonably clear purpose: description, exploration, tabulation, or decoration.
- ▸ Be closely integrated with the statistical and verbal descriptions of a data set.

(Tufte, 1983)

lines, and labels; the non-erasable core of a graphic and the non-redundant ink arranged in response to variation in the numbers represented) and the de-emphasis of "non-data ink" (such as the title, the abscissa, and the ordinate and their labels), while changing the data ink as the data change. Tufte cites two relevant aphorisms in his 1983 book: "For non-data ink, less is more; for data ink, less is a bore."

One of the best ways to apply these principles of graphical excellence is not simply to trim the volume of content but to present the information that has been selected as "small multiples." To do this, an instructor can look for information that can be grouped together. As each new multiple of knowledge is added, emphasis is then placed both on its difference from and its similarity to the previous multiple. This tactic helps link the separate pieces of information (Tufte, 1983, 1990).

Small multiples can apply not only to data graphics, but also to text and to pictures. By far, the most elegant visual examples of how to present data as small multiples come from Tufte's books, but a few useful and simple examples of organizing a presentation's data, text, and pictures as small multiples follow.

**Data**. In presenting data for a lecture, PowerPoint "builds" are a good way to emphasize "data ink" because the "non-data ink" portions do not change as the data are "built."

In Figure 1-1, all the data are shown simultaneously. The message is implicit in the graphic and it is possible for the viewer to figure out the message eventually by searching this visual as someone explains it. Even before the visual is shown, the message may be made explicit and more memorable by the presenter stating out loud that the upcoming **issue** is how long to wait for remission after treatment with Drug A. The **action** that will be proposed, to be taken if the participant is convinced by the data, is to treat longer before giving up on severely ill patients than on moderately ill patients. The reasoning for this action is that much of the remission of moderately ill patients occurs before 6 to 8 weeks of treatment, whereas much of the remission of severely ill patients occurs after that time. Finally, the presenter can mention in advance of showing the slide what the **benefit** will be to the participant of understanding the issue and taking the action.

This graphic can serve to enhance learning and integrate the new information into clinical practice. It does show that, for severely ill patients, it may be beneficial to consider not switching or stopping this drug before most of the patients are likely to remit, even though that may mean waiting for a long time (more than 4 months) for them to remit. These words can all be used by the presenter to describe the fully built slide (1-1A).

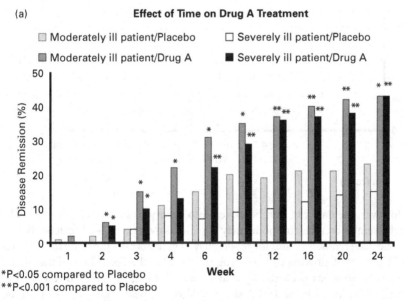

(a)    **Effect of Time on Drug A Treatment**

☐ Moderately ill patient/Placebo    ☐ Severely ill patient/Placebo
■ Moderately ill patient/Drug A    ■ Severely ill patient/Drug A

*P<0.05 compared to Placebo
**P<0.001 compared to Placebo

**Figure 1-1. Efficient use of data ink in slide presentations.** Panel A shows all data to be presented, while panels B–E present the information in a sequence of events.

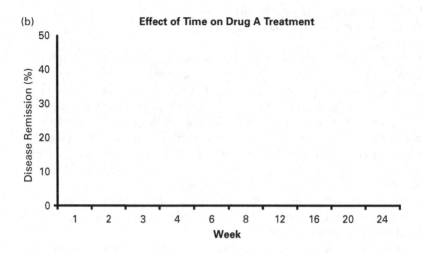

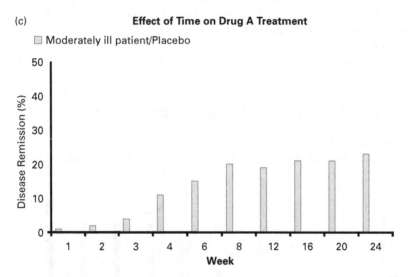

Figure 1-1. (cont.)

However, the data can also be woven into a story of small multiples. First the placebo remission rates for moderately ill patients over time (1-1B) can be shown, then the drug remission rates for moderately ill patients over the same time (1-1C) can be presented, proving that the drug works better than placebo and that much of the remission has occurred by 6 to 12 weeks. Next, the placebo rate for the severely ill patients can be added, showing lower placebo response than with the moderately ill patients (1-1D). The finale is the major point to be made, revealing drug remission rates for severely ill patients. The data in the finale show that, in

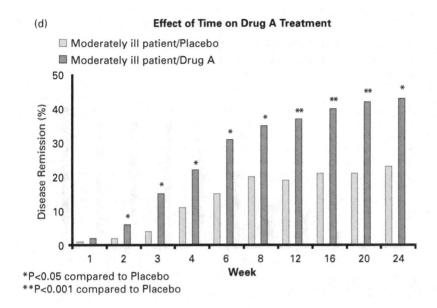

(d)

**Effect of Time on Drug A Treatment**

Moderately ill patient/Placebo
Moderately ill patient/Drug A

*P<0.05 compared to Placebo
**P<0.001 compared to Placebo

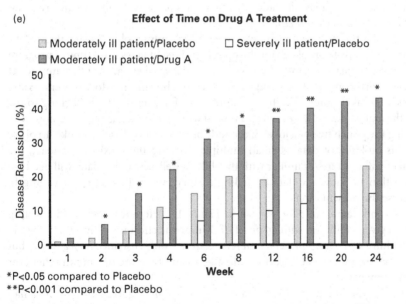

(e)

**Effect of Time on Drug A Treatment**

Moderately ill patient/Placebo          Severely ill patient/Placebo
Moderately ill patient/Drug A

*P<0.05 compared to Placebo
**P<0.001 compared to Placebo

Figure 1-1. (cont.)

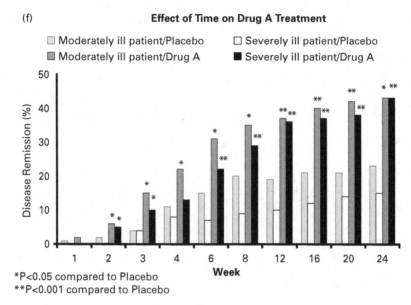

(f)                    **Effect of Time on Drug A Treatment**

☐ Moderately ill patient/Placebo      ☐ Severely ill patient/Placebo
■ Moderately ill patient/Drug A      ■ Severely ill patient/Drug A

*P<0.05 compared to Placebo
**P<0.001 compared to Placebo

Figure 1-1. (cont.)

contrast to moderately ill patients, many of the severely ill patients respond AFTER 6 to 12 weeks (1-1E).

Although this approach can be a powerful learning tool and behavioral motivator, it does create problems for the presenter. First, it takes extra time to program the builds. More importantly, however, is that the speaker has to anticipate and set up each forthcoming slide build in advance of showing it. Most presenters use slides as speaker notes, and this does not work for data building. Clicking to the end through slides 1-1B to 1-1E and then starting to speak has the same impact as putting the punch line of a joke on the slide before starting to tell the joke. In order for this building of data as small multiples to have the maximum impact, the speaker will want to be familiar with the slide as well as with the data, will need the motivation to show the data by telling a story, and will need to be willing to rehearse the presentation.

A second data example is shown in Figure 1-2. Here the story is that a drug treats a given condition with an onset of therapeutic effect not only within 1 week, but within 1 day. Drug–placebo differences are not only sustained for 12 weeks, but the effect size of drug at 2 weeks is already greater than the maximum relief ever attained by placebo.

These data can be presented all at once, as in Figure 1-2A, or in small multiples. The small multiples approach would begin with an explanation of the study design and what was measured, before any data are shown. Tufte refers to this practice as showing the non-data ink before showing the data ink. Since the non-data ink would not change for the next five builds, all the eye would see

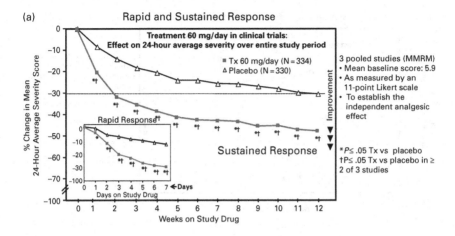

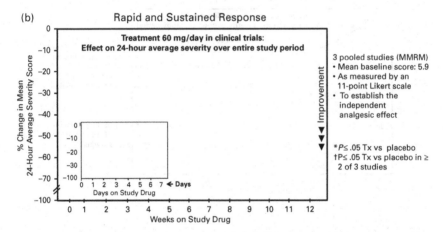

Figure 1-2. **Example of data ink in combination with small multiples.** Data can be presented all at once, as in Figure 1-2A or in small multiples, as in Figures 1-2B-G. Figure 1-2B shows only non-data ink, which does not change as data ink is added in the next five builds.

is the new information, including its relationship to the information already presented.

As the presenter clicks through these five builds, the presenter is exploiting an involuntary visual reflex. Anyone who has seen the data ink in Figure 1-2B has accommodated to it, and when the placebo group is added (Figure 1-2C), this causes the viewer to see how these data relate to the study design. There is no need for a laser pointer here. Also, if a computer screen is in front of the presenter, there is no need for the presenter to turn towards the screen and lose eye contact with the audience.

(c)

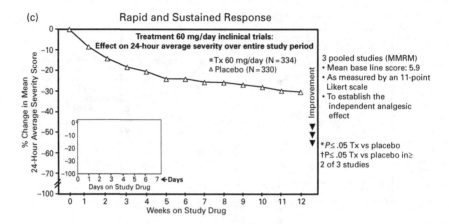

(d)

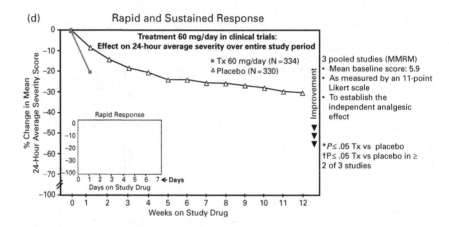

(e)

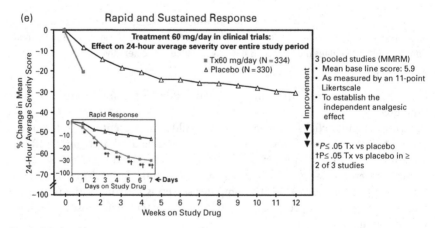

Figure 1-2. (cont.)

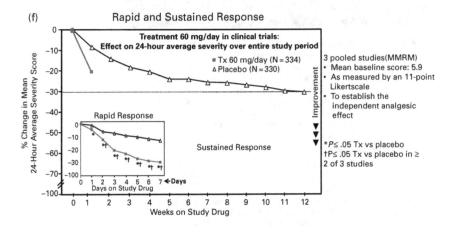

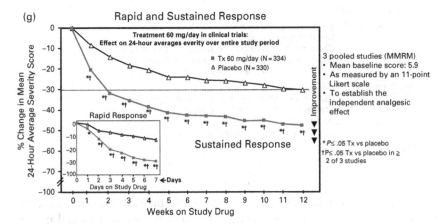

Figure 1-2. (cont.)

The next click (Figure 1-2D) shows the beginning of drug response. This is effective in emphasizing rapid onset of action due both to stopping the data at the first time point of 1 week and then exploding the first time point into an insert showing time points every day over the first week with the next click (Figure 1-2E).

Next, the presenter shows a target of drug efficacy to beat, namely the highest level of symptom relief caused by placebo, represented by the dashed horizontal line (Figure 1-2F). To finish, the presenter adds the coup de grace, namely, the rest of the time–response curve of drug, showing its relationship to placebo at each time point and to the end point of placebo (Figure 1-2G).

**Text.** Using small multiples of text allows the medical instructor to modulate the speed of learning. As in graphic presentations of data, animations of portions of

**TABLE 1-2:** Parallel structure in bullet points

| | |
|---|---|
| Before | Drug A: PROS<br>▸ Can be used off label for dementia with aggressive features<br>▸ Has been studied in children with various behavioral disturbances<br>▸ Long-acting form available that is useful for noncompliant patients<br>▸ Becoming generic soon and will be inexpensive |
| Sort by | After |
| Verbs | Benefits of Drug A<br>▸ Treats dementia with aggressive features (off label)<br>▸ Treats various behavioral disturbances in children (off label except autism)<br>▸ Treats noncompliant patients (long-acting formulation)<br>▸ Costs less than similar drugs (with generic soon available) |
| Sort by | After |
| Direct objects | Drug A is useful for treating<br>▸ Dementia with aggressive features<br>▸ Children with various behavioral disturbances<br>▸ Noncompliant patients (long-acting form)<br>▸ Financially restricted patients |
| Patient type and drug characteristics | Drug A treats<br>▸ Dementia with aggressive features<br>▸ Children with various behavioral disturbances<br>▸ At low cost<br>▸ In a long-acting formulation |
| (Stahl, 2009) | |

text can be used to make each multiple appear as the medical instructor speaks to that specific topic. In this way, learners move ahead with the instructor and are not distracted by coming information.

In text, presenting bullet points in parallel structure can help emphasize small multiples. To achieve parallel structure, the instructor can start each bullet with the same type of word: all verbs, all nouns, etc. Table 1-2 shows some examples of parallel structure.

Parallel structure is the way to separate data ink from non-data ink in a text slide. That is, the non-data ink is the structure of the words. If there is a parallel structure, there is no new structure to figure out with each new line of text, and the form of the words becomes non-data ink. That frees the reader to "see" only what is novel with each new bullet point, namely, the substance of the new information, i.e., the data ink. By the time there is a third bullet point, the pattern is established and it is progressively easier to get to the substance of subsequently developing text. An example of developing a slide with parallel structure and small multiples of text is shown in Figure 1-3.

(a)                     Drug A

– Can be used off label for dementia with aggressive features

– Has been studied in children with various behavioral disturbances

– Long-acting form available that is useful for noncompliant patients

– Becoming generic soon and will be inexpensive

– Elevates prolactin

– Weight gain (especially in children)

– Risk of stroke in elderly (especially with atrial fibrillation)

– May cause motor side effects (especially in patients with Parkinson's disease or Lewy body dementia)

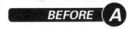

(b)         Drug A: Pros and Cons

> **PROS**
>
> – Treats dementia with aggressive features (off label)
>
> – Treats behavioral disturbances in children (off label except autism)
>
> – Treats noncompliant patients (long-acting formulation)
>
> – Becoming generic soon and will be inexpensive

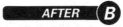

Figure 1-3. **Parceling out text slides into small multiples.** Each box could be made to appear individually using animations or builds. The corresponding pros and cons boxes have parallel structure and the multiples allow the audience to compare patients who would benefit with those who would not. Figure 1-3A shows all of the data. Figure 1-3B and C show that data in small multiples with parallel structure. (Stahl, 2009)

**Pictures.** Since small multiples resemble the frames of a movie, it is relatively easy to deconstruct the figure of a dynamic biological process into its "stop action" components as the process proceeds from beginning to end. Of course, Flash animations can do this continuously and smoothly but are even

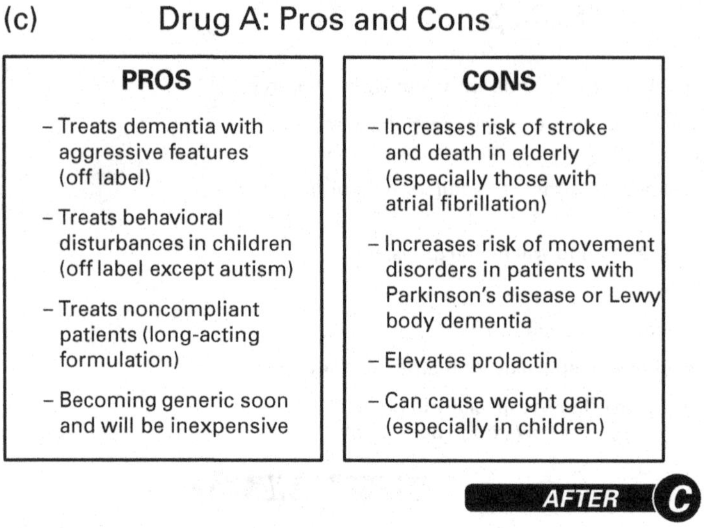

(c)             Drug A: Pros and Cons

| PROS | CONS |
|------|------|
| – Treats dementia with aggressive features (off label) | – Increases risk of stroke and death in elderly (especially those with atrial fibrillation) |
| – Treats behavioral disturbances in children (off label except autism) | – Increases risk of movement disorders in patients with Parkinson's disease or Lewy body dementia |
| – Treats noncompliant patients (long-acting formulation) | – Elevates prolactin |
| – Becoming generic soon and will be inexpensive | – Can cause weight gain (especially in children) |

AFTER  **C**

Figure 1-3. (cont.)

more time-consuming to develop than PowerPoint builds. If successful, this PowerPoint display tactic will draw attention entirely to shifts in the data and thus to what is happening next in a sequence of actions. This tactic also exploits the same involuntary visual reflex as discussed previously for data graphics. The eye will go to the new or changed elements – those that are appearing, disappearing, or moving. The eye will also see the relationship of these elements to the non-data ink components that came before.

Small multiple displays (see Table 1-3) can also show causality among various parameters such as:
● before and after (surgery, medication, activation, etc.)
● with and without
● young versus old
● healthy versus diseased

An example of this is shown in Figure 1-4. One way to build this is to show everything on the same slide, as illustrated in Figures 1-4A through 1-4F. Another is to superimpose the images upon each other sequentially, as shown in Figures 1-4G through 1-4M. The advantage of the first tactic is that it is easier to review the entire build. The advantage of the second tactic is that there is less non-data ink and thus more emphasis on what is changing dynamically, as well as the relationship of these changes to what has come before in the sequence. Either tactic is acceptable and better than a complex slide with no builds.

The point of Figure 1-4 is to show that the amygdala processes the emotion of fear and that the more fear processing there is, the more prone one is to anxiety.

(a)            A Fear-Related Stimulus Causes Amygdalar
              Overactivation in Carriers of the "Short" SERT

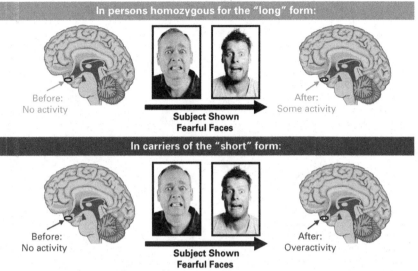

Stahl SM. *Stahl's Essential Psychopharmacology.* 3rd ed. 2008.

Figure 1-4. **Parceling out image slides into small multiples.** The "before" slide (Figure 1-4A) presents all of the information at once, which may be overwhelming and therefore have low impact. In the "after" slides (Figures 1-4B–F), the parceling out allows the instructor to use PowerPoint builds to bring information in slowly.

- Under the top half of the figure, the "long"/before condition could be shown and explained; then the stimulus presented; and then the "long"/after condition revealed.
- Under the bottom half of the figure, the "short"/before condition could be shown; then the stimulus presented; and then the "short"/after condition revealed.
  Other examples of this principle follow in Figures 1-4G–M. (Stahl, 2008)

Furthermore, there is one genotype of the serotonin transporter that creates greater reactivity of emotional processing in the amygdala than another genotype and thus carries a greater risk of an anxiety disorder than another. All this can be said in a complex, complete version of the slide (Figure 1-4A). However, the story can be developed by first showing the non-data ink with the title, the subtitles, and two identical brains with no activity. One of these brains is in a person with the first genotype and the other is in a person with the second genotype (Figure 1-4B). When one builds the provocation of fear by showing a scary face while the subject is in the brain scanner (Figures 1-4C and 1-4E), then one can set up the low activation of the amygdala in those with the first genotype (Figure 1-4D) but the high activation of the amygdala in those with the second genotype, who respond with a high degree of amygdala activation (Figure 1-4F).

(b)    A Fear-Related Stimulus Causes Amygdalar
Overactivation in Carriers of the "Short" SERT

**In persons homozygous for the "long" form:**

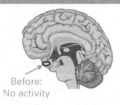

Before:
No activity

**In carriers of the "short" form:**

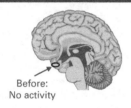

Before:
No activity

Stahl SM. *Stahl's Essential Psychopharmacology.* 3$^{rd}$ ed. 2008.

(c)    A Fear-Related Stimulus Causes Amygdalar
Overactivation in Carriers of the "Short" SERT

**In persons homozygous for the "long" form:**

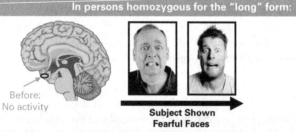

Before:
No activity

**Subject Shown
Fearful Faces**

**In carriers of the "short" form:**

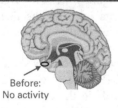

Before:
No activity

Stahl SM. *Stahl's Essential Psychopharmacology.* 3$^{rd}$ ed. 2008.

Figure 1-4. (cont.)

(d)             A Fear-Related Stimulus Causes Amygdalar
                Overactivation in Carriers of the "Short" SERT

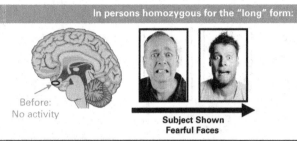

Stahl SM. *Stahl's Essential Psychopharmacology.* 3$^{rd}$ ed. 2008.

(e)             A Fear-Related Stimulus Causes Amygdalar
                Overactivation in Carriers of the "Short" SERT

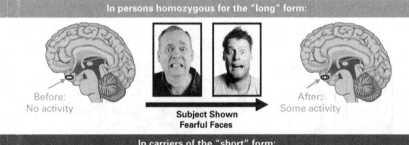

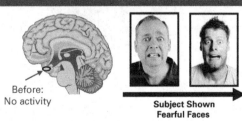

Stahl SM. *Stahl's Essential Psychopharmacology.* 3$^{rd}$ ed. 2008.

**Figure 4-1. (cont.)**

(f)    A Fear-Related Stimulus Causes Amygdalar
Overactivation in Carriers of the "Short" SERT

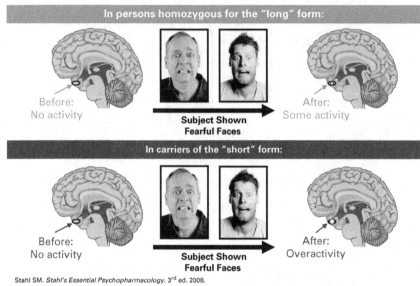

Stahl SM. *Stahl's Essential Psychopharmacology.* 3$^{rd}$ ed. 2008.

(g)    Neuroimaging the Functional Consequences of a
Subtle Molecular Abnormality in SERT Part 1: l/l Variants of SERT

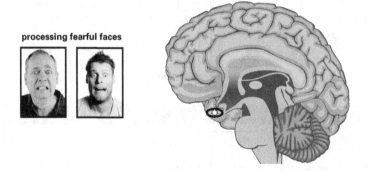

Stahl SM. *Stahl's Essential Psychopharmacology.* 3$^{rd}$ ed. 2008.

**Figure 1-4. (cont.)**

(h)    Neuroimaging the Functional Consequences of a
Subtle Molecular Abnormality in SERT
Part 1: l/l Variants of SERT

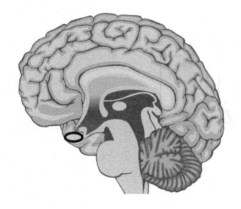

Stahl SM. *Stahl's Essential Psychopharmacology.* 3$^{rd}$ ed. 2008.

(i)    Neuroimaging the Functional Consequences of a
Subtle Molecular Abnormality in SERT
Part 1: l/l Variants of SERT

**processing fearful faces**

     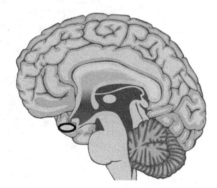

Stahl SM. *Stahl's Essential Psychopharmacology.* 3$^{rd}$ ed. 2008.

**Figure 1-4. (cont.)**

(j)          Neuroimaging the Functional Consequences of a
              Subtle Molecular Abnormality in SERT
                    Part 1: I/I Variants of SERT

**processing fearful faces**

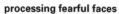

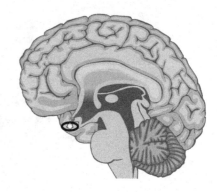

Stahl SM. *Stahl's Essential Psychopharmacology.* 3$^{rd}$ ed. 2008.

(k)                        Part 2:
                      S Carriers of SERT

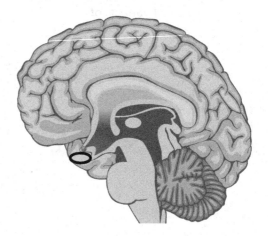

Stahl SM. *Stahl's Essential Psychopharmacology.* 3$^{rd}$ ed. 2008.

**Figure 1-4. (cont.)**

(l)

Part 2:
S Carriers of SERT

**processing fearful faces**

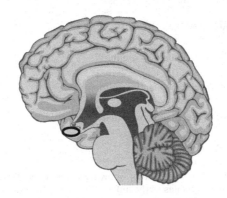

Stahl SM. *Stahl's Essential Psychopharmacology.* 3<sup>rd</sup> ed. 2008.

(m)

Part 2:
S Carriers of SERT

**processing fearful faces**

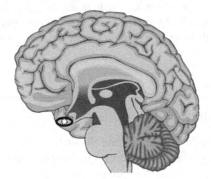

Stahl SM. *Stahl's Essential Psychopharmacology.* 3<sup>rd</sup> ed. 2008.

**Figure 1-4. (cont.)**

One can also show this by superimposing the figures (Figures 1-4G through 1-4M). This eliminates a great deal of "non-data ink" and works much better in PowerPoint than in print.

Table 1-3 gives a review of how to use well-designed small multiples for an effective presentation.

**TABLE 1-3**: Review of the characteristics of presentations using well-designed small multiples

- ▸ Inevitably comparable multiples

- ▸ Deftly multivariate

- ▸ Shrunken, high-density graphics

- ▸ Usually based on a large data matrix

- ▸ Drawn almost entirely with data ink

- ▸ Efficient in interpretation

- ▸ Often narrative in content, showing shifts in the relationship between variables as the index variable changes (thereby revealing interactions or multiplicative effects)

(Tufte,1983)

### Section summary: organizing content as small multiples

Delivering information in small multiples gives learners manageable packets of information and helps them to see the differences and similarities between conditions, deepening their understanding of what was presented (see Stahl and Davis 2009b).

## Section 3

### Visual additions

Surveys in adult education have shown that instructors tend to labor over instructional and conceptual features, but learners tend to focus on surface attributes, such as appearance (Price, 2007). More specifically, learners prefer visual representations to text-heavy materials (Price, 2007). In fact, the majority of adults (up to 75%) are visual learners or visual-multimodal learners (Baykan and Nacar, 2007). Visual learners focus on the illustrative elements of presentations, such as diagrams, symbols, graphs, flow charts, hierarchies, figures, and models. Therefore, visual representations incorporated into presentations will aid in their learning process.

Adding visual representations does not mean using clip art, fancy backgrounds, or three-dimensional effects on charts. The goal is to increase learning, not detract from it or decorate it. Medical education is a visually rich field; many images and figures representing anatomy and pharmacology are readily available. In addition, live presentations offer a freedom of space that is unavailable in journals and other publications. Proper use of space can help to translate textual information into visual representations. Can a text-heavy description be translated into a visually clear figure? Can a numbers-only table be converted into a bar chart or line graph? Instructors may want to translate a text description into a figure (Figure 1-5). A text-based table may be turned into a chart in which bars stand out obviously (Figure 1-6) so learners are not forced to hunt for important statistics and differences.

Data visuals can also be combined with pictures (Figure 1-6). Thus, another powerful visual tactic is to show data simultaneously with a pictorial representation of the same data in another form. This causes a highly impactful visual correlation and a hard-to-forget lesson on the relationships between the data and the picture.

## Section summary: visual additions

Because so many audience members prefer visual components in their learning materials, including relevant images and figures, wherever reasonable, can increase the learning impact of the presentation and aid the effectiveness of the instructor.

## Section 4

### Applying principles of multimedia learning

When used properly, modern instructional tools offer many opportunities to increase the educational impact of a presentation. This section examines some principles established by Richard Mayer, a researcher in multimedia learning (see BioBox 1-2) to guide the use of multimedia instruction.

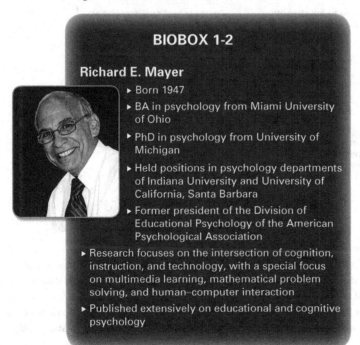

**BIOBOX 1-2**

**Richard E. Mayer**

- Born 1947
- BA in psychology from Miami University of Ohio
- PhD in psychology from University of Michigan
- Held positions in psychology departments of Indiana University and University of California, Santa Barbara
- Former president of the Division of Educational Psychology of the American Psychological Association
- Research focuses on the intersection of cognition, instruction, and technology, with a special focus on multimedia learning, mathematical problem solving, and human–computer interaction
- Published extensively on educational and cognitive psychology

(a)     Dosing Strategies for Switching Drugs

| Delayed Withdrawal | Cross-Titration |
|---|---|
| • Strategy: Add second drug to full strength before decreasing first drug | • Strategy: Decrease first drug somewhat before increasing second drug |
| • PRO: Beneficial when relapse is a concern | • PRO: Beneficial for stable patients experiencing side effects |
| • CON: Potential for increased side effects | • CON: Possible disease breakthrough due to sub-therapeutic doses of both agents |

**BEFORE**

(b)     Dosing Strategies for Switching Drugs

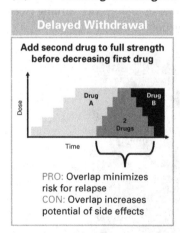
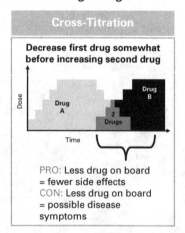

**AFTER**

Figure 1-5. **Translating a text slide into a visual slide.**

The "before" slide is a good start – the information is parceled out to allow the learner to compare the two strategies. However, it does not use visual representations, and it does not show cause and effect (differences in dosing affecting efficacy and tolerability).

To achieve the "after" slide, dosing strategies were given a visual representation, and items were grouped into "cause" (dosing strategy, green overlap) and "effect" (green boxes). (Stahl, 2008)

(a)
## Reproductive Contrasts:
## Hunter-Gatherers Versus Modern Americans

|  | Hunter-Gatherers | Modern Americans |
|---|---|---|
| Age at menarche (y) | 16.1 | 12.5 |
| Number of pregnancies | 5.9 | 1.8 |
| Duration of breastfeeding per birth (mo) | 35 | 3 |
| Estimated number of menstrual cycles | 160 | 450 |

Eaton SB, *et al.* Q Rev Biol. 1994;69:353-367.     **BEFORE**

(b)
## Reproductive Contrasts:
## Hunter-Gatherers Versus Modern Americans

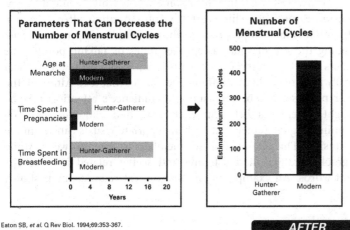

Eaton SB, *et al.* Q Rev Biol. 1994;69:353-367.     **AFTER**

Figure 1-6. **Converting a table to a visual representation.**
- The "before" slide is a good start – the information is parceled out to allow the learner to compare the two kinds of women. However, it does not use visual representations, and it does not show cause and effect (changes in reproductive patterns leading to more menstrual cycles).
- To achieve the visual representation in the "after" slide
  - Items were grouped into "cause" (left box) and "effect" (right box)
  - "Cause" items were made parallel ("before" uses three different units – years, number, and months – but "after" shows all items translated into years)
  - Table/text numbers were presented as bars, with size indicating value

(Eaton, 1994)

### The modality principle

Different audience members may prefer different learning styles, but most have a preference for multimodal learning. Beyond preferences, results-oriented research has shown that information should be encoded both visually and auditorily to increase learning (Mayer, 2001). There may be concern that two competing sources of information could overwhelm or overload the learner. However, adult working memory has two somewhat independent subcomponents that tend to work in parallel, allowing learners to process information simultaneously coming from their eyes and their ears. This is called dual coding. Thus, learners are not overwhelmed or overloaded by multimodal instruction; instead, learning is enhanced when information is presented both auditorily and visually as long as the inputs are synchronized and mutually reinforcing, rather than competing inputs of different information in one modality versus another or, at worst, conflicting inputs (Mayer, 2001).

### The redundancy principle

According to this principle, students learn better from a combination of simple visuals plus simultaneous auditory narration than from visuals plus added on-screen text combined with simultaneous auditory narration (Mayer, 2001). Audiences do not learn well when they hear some words while seeing different words with the same message. This creates a split-attention effect. From a learning standpoint, it is most appropriate to eliminate redundant text material while also avoiding the use of slides as speaker notes or talking points. The audience members may be reading what is written on-screen while the medical instructor verbally presents a slightly different version of that text. Although the basic concept or premise may be the same, the audience's attention may be diverted by slight differences between what is written and what is said. Replacing or minimizing on-screen text with appropriate visuals can eliminate this type of confusion. This allows audience members to listen to words while looking at a graphic, rather than listening and seeing related but perhaps slightly different words. An example of eliminating text redundancy is shown in Figure 1-7.

### The contiguity principles (spatial and temporal)

The pairing of learning elements in both time and space is important. Students learn better when corresponding words and pictures are presented in close proximity rather than far from each other on the page or screen (Mayer, 2001). Similarly, students learn better when corresponding words and pictures are presented simultaneously rather than successively (Mayer, 2001). Thus, good slide design calls for visually pairing elements in a common pattern.

To link further these two types of media, the proper use of builds can be employed by making paired information appear together, as shown in Figure 1-8.

(a)    Norepinephrine (NE) and Depression Symptoms

- Norepinephrine-containing cells in the locus coeruleus of the brainstem innervate and affect many brain regions associated with symptoms of depression
- Relationships between NE and symptoms of depression:
  - dorsolateral prefrontal cortex associated with problems concentrating
  - hypothalamus associated with trouble sleeping (hypersomnia or insomnia) and change in weight or appetite
  - amygdala associated with anxious symptoms
  - cerebellum associated with physical fatigue
  - NE mediates incoming pain signals in spinal cord; may explain somatic complaints

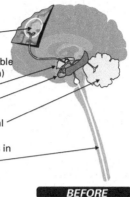

Stahl SM. Stahl's Essential Psychopharmacology. 3rd ed. 2008.

**BEFORE**

(b)                    Norepinephrine and Depression Symptoms

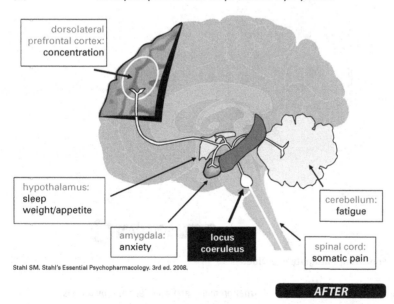

Stahl SM. Stahl's Essential Psychopharmacology. 3rd ed. 2008.

**AFTER**

Figure 1-7. **Eliminating textual redundancy in a slide.** The "before" slide has almost every word the instructor intends to say written out on the slide. The "after" slide has whittled down that same information to just one or two reminder words. (Stahl, 2008)

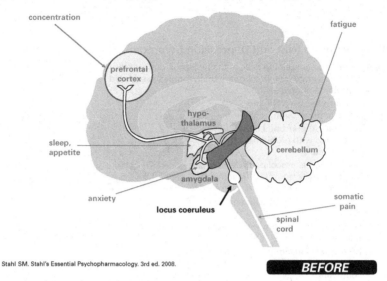

(a) Norepinephrine and Depression Symptoms

concentration

fatigue

prefrontal cortex

hypo-thalamus

sleep, appetite

cerebellum

amygdala

anxiety

**locus coeruleus**

somatic pain

spinal cord

Stahl SM. Stahl's Essential Psychopharmacology. 3rd ed. 2008.

**BEFORE**

(b) Norepinephrine and Depression Symptoms

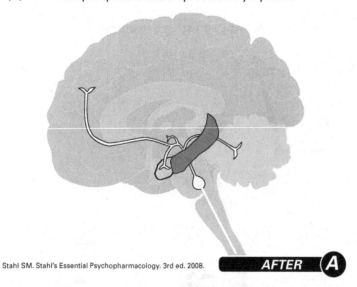

Stahl SM. Stahl's Essential Psychopharmacology. 3rd ed. 2008.

**AFTER** **A**

Figure 1-8 **Enhancing contiguity in a slide.**

Spatial

- The "before" slide shows the information pairs separated far apart by arrows.
- The "after" slides visually bring the symptom and its anatomy closer together.

Temporal

- Contiguity in the "before" slide would be reduced by using builds to explain first the anatomy and then the symptomatology. This would temporally separate each symptom from its corresponding anatomical location.
- Contiguity in the "after" slides would be enhanced by using builds to make the text in each box appear together. For example, the words *amygdala* and *anxiety* could be made to appear with one click; this build would enhance their temporal contiguity.

(Stahl, 2008)

(c)         Norepinephrine and Depression Symptoms

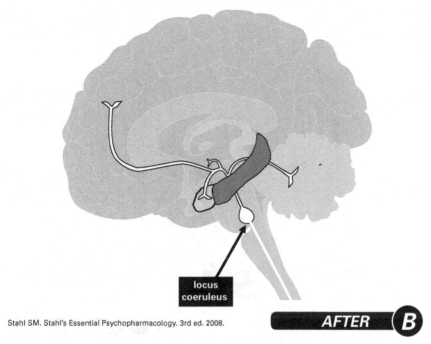

locus
coeruleus

AFTER   **B**

(d)         Norepinephrine and Depression Symptoms

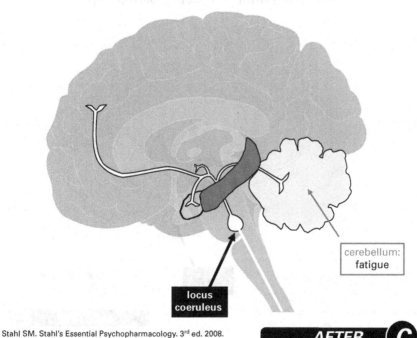

locus
coeruleus

cerebellum:
fatigue

AFTER   **C**

Figure 1-8. (cont.)

(e)              Norepinephrine and Depression Symptoms

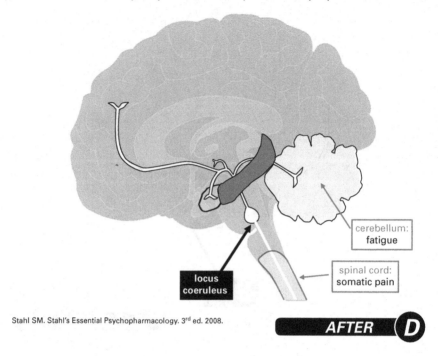

cerebellum:
fatigue

spinal cord:
somatic pain

locus
coeruleus

Stahl SM. Stahl's Essential Psychopharmacology. 3rd ed. 2008.

AFTER  D

(f)              Norepinephrine and Depression Symptoms

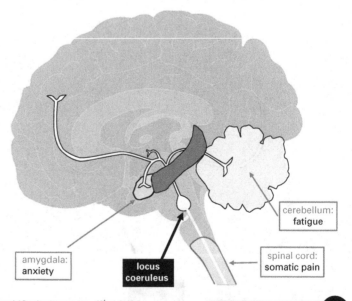

cerebellum:
fatigue

amygdala:
anxiety

locus
coeruleus

spinal cord:
somatic pain

Stahl SM. Stahl's Essential Psychopharmacology. 3rd ed. 2008.

AFTER  E

Figure 1-8. (cont.)

(g)    Norepinephrine and Depression Symptoms

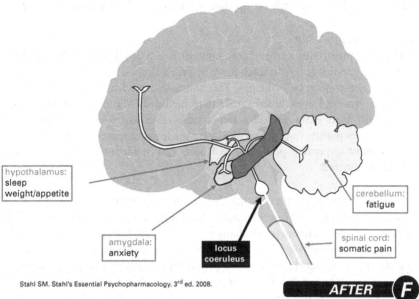

Stahl SM. Stahl's Essential Psychopharmacology. 3rd ed. 2008.

(h)    Norepinephrine and Depression Symptoms

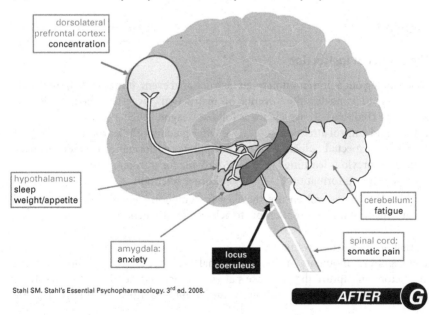

Stahl SM. Stahl's Essential Psychopharmacology. 3rd ed. 2008.

Figure 1-8 (cont.)

While legends are common elements in medical presentations, they break up the spatial contiguity of slides. Whenever possible, legends can be eliminated and labels can be put directly on the data. An example is shown in Figure 1-9.

### The coherence principle

As has been mentioned earlier, more content is not always better. It may be a cliché, but sometimes one can teach more by presenting less. This is more formally known as the coherence principle. This states that students learn more when extraneous material is excluded rather than included (Mayer, 2001). Padding a presentation with extra material can actually decrease learning rather than strengthen key points. In order to maximize the learning potential of a presentation, the most important points on each slide can be identified and extraneous material eliminated.

### Section summary: applying principles of multimedia learning

To increase the impact of presentations, information can be presented in both auditory and visual channels (modality principle); interference from the textual channel can be eliminated (redundancy principle); related information can be presented in close spatial and temporal proximity (contiguity principles); and key topics can be identified and extraneous information eliminated (coherence principle). When followed, these principles will create a platform that sets up the instructor to convey key messages to the audience and to raise his or her effectiveness as a medical instructor and facilitator.

## Section 5

### The events of instruction

When laying out a presentation or an instructional event, it may be helpful for the instructor to consider the "events of instruction" as established by Robert M. Gagné (BioBox 1-3), which are as follows (Gagné, 1965):

1. Gain and control attention
2. Describe expected outcomes
3. Refer to previous learning
4. Present new information

5. Offer guidance for learning
6. Appraise performance/provide feedback
7. Provide for transferability
8. Ensure retention

These guidelines will ensure that key presentation elements are not omitted when a medical instructor attempts to achieve an instructional goal.

### 1. Gain and control attention

The beginning moments of an instructional event are especially important. An instructor can capture the audience's attention more efficiently by first resolving distractions that arise from tensions in the learning environment. (This principle

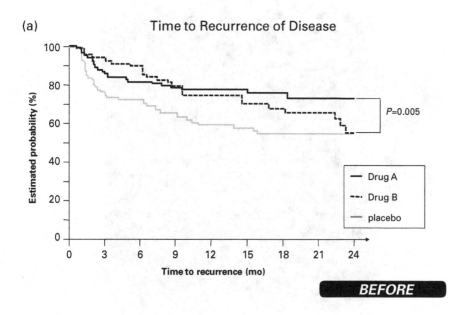

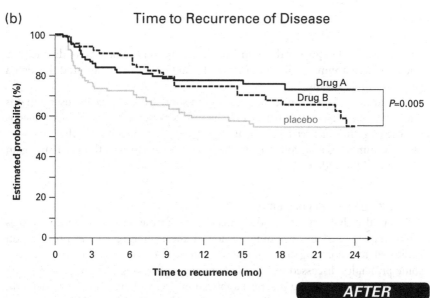

Figure 1-9. **Removing a legend to increase contiguity.** Spatially, legends can be incorporated into a figure or table not only to create a more visibly appealing learning tool but also to reduce distraction by providing information in a more relevant location when compared to presented data. (Keller et al., 2007)

**BIOBOX 1-3**

**Robert Mills Gagné**

- 1916–2002
- BA from Yale University; PhD in experimental psychology from Brown University
- Research director at the perceptual and motor skills laboratory of the US Air Force
- Professorships in psychology and educational psychology at Connecticut College for Women; Pennsylvania State University; Princeton University; University of California, Berkeley; and Florida State University
- Published extensively on instructional theory and design
- Work influenced American education system as well as military and industrial training

will be discussed in greater detail in Chapter 2.) Beyond resolution of distractions due to the environment, the attention of the audience can be captured through a variety of other means.

One strategy is for the instructor to show a short video clip (a "focuser") that is relevant to the presentation before information is presented. Already mentioned is the use of a clinical anecdote, which also serves as an opening for the "three-act play." A humorous anecdote can also be quite effective to start things off and gain attention of the audience.

## 2. Describe expected outcomes

This has already been discussed in this chapter in the section on previews. It is often implemented by including a slide at the beginning of the presentation dedicated to informing the learners of expected outcomes. This also satisfies some principles discussed in this book: namely, providing a preview of learning to come and emphasizing practical application (to be discussed in more detail in Chapter 2). One arena of medical education with a good grasp of this concept is continuing medical education (CME), which requires that a CME provider give learning objectives that "communicate the purpose or objectives of the activity so the learner is informed before participating in the activity" (ACCME, 2008). Learning objectives designed with this approach typically start with a sentence like, "This presentation will show you how . . ." followed by a bulleted list of action goals using verbs such as the following:

- To diagnose
- To explain
- To define
- To understand

- To organize
- To prescribe
- To predict
- To solve

- To contrast
- To demonstrate
- To recognize
- To perform

Beyond use in one-off presentations, this guideline is also applicable to a lecture series or semester-long coursework. Long-term goals can be clearly stated at the beginning of the series while short-term goals can be provided at the beginning of each lecture.

## 3. Refer to previous learning

The first section or first few slides of a presentation can be designed to stimulate audience recall of relevant prerequisite capabilities and previous learning (Gagné, 1965). This is directly related to the principle, "draw on audience experience," discussed in more detail in Chapter 2. When it is time to introduce a new therapeutic option or topic, the instructor can first discuss older therapies that are familiar to the audience. When introducing new diagnostic criteria, an instructor can refer to older paradigms in which the audience is well versed. When introducing a simple concept, the instructor may find that "recognition" may be a sufficient referral to previous learning (e.g. "You all know about inhibitors of angiotensin-converting enzyme. Now, we will learn about . . ."). However, introducing more complex rules may require the "reinstatement" of previous learnings (e.g. in this particular case, an in-depth review of angiotensin-converting enzyme inhibitors might be appropriate).

In a series of lectures, compared to just a single presentation, the first lecture is a good opportunity to review prerequisite learning or established knowledge to provide a foundation from which the audience can work. As the series continues, a cumulative review of preceding material can be included in each successive lecture. This approach conforms to the concept of previews and reviews, discussed earlier in this chapter.

## 4. Present new information

Once the stage has been set with the preliminary events of instruction, the audience members will be prepared and maximally receptive, allowing them to focus their attention on receiving key messages provided by the medical instructor.

## 5. Offer guidance for learning

Guidance for learning may take a variety of forms, depending on the format and goals of a talk. During the presentation, a medical instructor can guide learning by asking questions that stimulate the learner to discover rules and principles. For instance, when teaching learners that the side effect of a drug is nausea, the medical instructor could say, "Since you know that this drug can stimulate peripheral serotonin receptors in the gut, what side effects might you expect a patient to report when first taking this medication?" After the presentation, worksheets, such as printouts of the slides with words omitted for fill-in-the-blank exercises, can be distributed to guide learning, allowing audience members to "discover" key topics from the presentation on their own. Homework exercises are common examples of guidance for learning. Alternatively, this stimulus may come from a referral, during the presentation, to related resources such as prescribing information, Web sites, or journal articles.

### 6. Appraise performance/provide feedback

During a learning event, learners must be able to perceive the results of their progress. Ideally, feedback will be provided that enables learners to realize whether their learning is correct – and that potentially also allows the medical instructor to make on-the-fly adjustments. In a long-term learning series, this criterion is typically fulfilled with quizzes or exams. Even in a one-off presentation, audience response questions using keypads can be included, as will be discussed later in this chapter. Evaluations by the instructor or graded exams are not always necessary, but at the minimum this tactic can provide a way for learners to assess their own performance.

### 7. Provide for transferability

Once an intellectual skill has been acquired, it needs to be put to use or it is likely to be forgotten. True learning involves more than understanding a principle; it means being able to apply the principle in novel situations. Case studies are particularly helpful in providing for transferability within presentations, especially in the medical field. In order to continue this learning process after the presentation is over, it may be valuable to provide resources that help learners use newly acquired information. This can be accomplished, for example, by the distribution of prescribing information, clinical trial data, anatomical posters, or slides and by encouraging learners to review relevant sections with a patient when prescribing a new medication or diagnosing a new condition.

### 8. Ensure retention

This criterion, though listed separately, actually encompasses many of the other criteria – perhaps even all of them. Enhancing learner retention can be accomplished with fulfillment of each of the criteria previously discussed.

### Section summary: the events of instruction

To increase the impact of presentations or learning events, information can be presented in accordance with the events of instruction: gain and control attention, describe expected outcomes, and refer to previous learning – all before new information or the next topic is presented. After summarizing a section or topic, the medical instructor can then offer guidance for learning, appraise performance or provide feedback, and provide for transferability. Together, these events of instruction help ensure learner retention of the presented material. Table 1-4 summarizes how the principles discussed in this chapter thus far can be applied to the effective design of slide sets.

**TABLE 1-4:** Checklist for designing a slide set

| Item | Rationale |
|---|---|
| Opening Sections | Opportunity to: |
| ☐ Optional: starts with a video clip? Or a question? Or a case study? | Gain and control attention Encourage involvement |
| ☐ Contains an outline slide? | Preview and review |
| ☐ Contains a learning objectives slide? | Describe expected outcomes Provide structure |
| ☐ Contains pretest questions? | Add questions for audience feedback Challenge |
| ☐ Refers to previous learning? | Refer to previous learning Challenge |
| Content Sections | |
| ☐ Text and images parceled into small multiples | Small multiples |
| ☐ Contains visual translations? | Visual additions Modality principle |
| ☐ Text minimized on slides? | Redundancy principle |
| ☐ Related information in close proximity? | Contiguity principle |
| ☐ Extra material eliminated or minimized? | Coherence principle |
| ☐ Reviews at end of every section? | Preview and review |
| Closing Sections | Opportunity for: |
| ☐ Contains posttest questions? | Feedback, appraising performance/providing feedback Adding questions for audience feedback |
| ☐ Integrates new information with previous learning? | Integration |
| ☐ Offers opportunity for practical application, such as case study? | Transferability Application |

## Section 6

### The conditions of learning

Another well-established paradigm for instructional design is the "conditions of learning" (Blocher, 1974). This model suggests that providing the audience with all of the following is necessary for optimizing learning and retention:

1. Involvement     5. Feedback
2. Challenge       6. Application
3. Support         7. Integration
4. Structure

## 1. Involvement

This parameter suggests that the learners need to put their values and beliefs at risk in order to entertain new learning (Blocher, 1974). In presentation situations, the audience members believe in and value their ability to be competent physicians. Therefore, calling that self-concept into question can help jump-start audience members and get them involved in the learning process. One way to fulfill this criterion is to use "focusers" to invest audience members emotionally in the learning activities. For example, presenting a video of a patient affected by a relevant disorder, while prompting learners to evaluate their confidence in and ability to help that patient, can emotionally engage audience members, making them more interested in the discussion about to take place.

## 2. Challenge

This parameter suggests that old learning needs to be challenged by novelty, complexity, ambiguity, and intensity (Blocher, 1974). This is similar to the "refer to previous learning" event previously discussed. By referring to the audience's knowledge base, the instructor can challenge assumptions. For example, an instructor could open with a discussion of a medication or a procedure that is the traditional first-line therapy and then suggest reasons that this usual strategy might be suboptimal.

## 3. Support

This parameter suggests that new learning needs an environment of empathy, caring, and honesty (Blocher, 1974), both from other learners and from the instructor. Instructors need to be open to questions from the audience, and dealing with questions appropriately can ensure that learners feel supported. The finer points associated with this paradigm and a few tactics to address these issues will be discussed in Chapter 2.

## 4. Structure

This parameter suggests that learners must understand what is to be done and how, similar to the "describe expected outcomes" condition reviewed earlier in this chapter. Moreover, it has been suggested that learning can be enhanced by designing an environment that models slightly more advanced structures than the old learning (Blocher, 1974). To explain further, if a new learning event is superior to the conditions under which the audience learned their previous beliefs, they will value the information, presentation, and instructor more than the educational experience they received earlier.

## 5. Feedback

As discussed earlier, learners need the opportunity to try out new learning modes in the presence of accurate and immediate information about their performance (Blocher, 1974). If the audience members receive no feedback or opportunity to evaluate their own learning, they will not value the information they receive as highly.

## 6. Application

The learners need ways to try out their new skills (Blocher, 1974). Inclusion of an activity that tests and requires learners to practice new skills, such as a case study, is a great application medium for health care providers, as they are already experienced with this type of learning technique. This principle is also in accordance with the earlier rule, "provide for transferability."

## 7. Integration

Learners need to examine new learning and reconcile it with past experiences (Blocher, 1974). At the end of a presentation, the instructor may want to come full circle, returning to the "old" paradigms that were used to open the lecture. Helping the learners see how new information fits with previous concepts achieves knowledge integration and allows audience members to reconcile both ideas for use in the future. For example, members of the audience may have experience with using a specific surgical approach to treating cancer but this may be presented with a slight variation, different technique, or newer technology for use in a very different disease state. The presentation could then end with a compare-and-contrast of the two techniques, followed by two case studies in which both options are relevant but one may be more beneficial in each case. Such an approach helps the audience members to integrate past information of the treatment with new knowledge in imagining a future application.

### Section summary: the conditions of learning

To increase the impact of presentations or educational events, information can be given in accordance with the "conditions of learning": learners should be involved and invested in learning; learners should be challenged on their current knowledge; an environment should be created that is supportive to the audience; a logical format and structure should be provided; opportunities for practical application should be offered; and learners should be given an opportunity to integrate previous learning with new information.

## Section 7

### Questions for audience feedback

Providing learners with feedback or the opportunity for self-evaluation of their learning is extremely important. An excellent approach to meeting this need is the use of an audience response system (ARS) to pose questions based on information presented. In collegiate settings, these systems are also called "student response systems," "personal response systems," or "classroom communication systems."

These response systems allow the instructor to ask questions on-screen at strategic moments in the presentation. Learners are then able to choose a response to questions by pressing a button on the response unit (or "keypad"), sending answers to the presentation computer. These personal response units vary in size – from as small as a credit card to as large as a television remote – and most have buttons labeled from 0 through 9. The response system receiver, which connects to the presentation computer, captures responses from students' keypads and shows the results on-screen.

If ARS technology is unavailable, a medical instructor can still pose questions to the audience and ask for a show of hands in response to each question. However, this visible response does have some drawbacks compared to an actual ARS system, as will be discussed.

## Benefits of audience response system questions

ARS questions:

- **Improve attentiveness and increase learning:** a survey of four University of Wisconsin campuses revealed that a majority of the 27 faculty respondents and the 2,684 student respondents agreed or strongly agreed that ARS keypads made learners more engaged in class and were beneficial to learning (Kaleta and Joosten, 2007).
- **Poll anonymously:** unlike a show of hands, responses by handheld keypad can be completely anonymous. This provides a learning environment that feels supportive, which is especially needed by some personality types.
- **Track individual and group responses:** response systems can be used to gather information about learning from each respondent and from the audience as a whole.
- **Gauge audience understanding:** in the University of Wisconsin survey mentioned above, 100% of the faculty respondents either agreed or strongly agreed with the claim, "Keypads allowed me to assess student knowledge on a particular concept" (Kaleta and Joosten, 2007). Students also recognized this benefit for their own self-assessment. Of student respondents, 75% agreed or strongly agreed with the claim, "Keypads helped me get instant feedback on what I knew and didn't know." By revealing to the instructor the level of understanding in the audience, ARS questions can help the instructor address and resolve confusion immediately.
- **Add interactivity and fun:** the novelty and interactivity of response systems can add interest to the learning environment. Respondents can even be grouped into teams (such as being divided by the two sides of the room), and team responses can be plotted against each other on the response screen. This adds a competitive gaming element to learning.

- **Evaluate participant learning:** structuring pretest questions prior to presenting the relevant material and posting test questions afterwards is one of the most efficient ways of measuring learning. Questions should be sufficiently difficult that everyone does not know the correct answer prior to the lecture, yet sufficiently easy so that learners can demonstrate new learning by pre–post comparisons.
- **Evaluate instructor teaching:** measuring learning gains of different lecturers against their ARS keypad questions can show whether the audience learned one section as well as another. Also, in situations where the same materials are presented to similar audiences but by different instructors, ARS questions with pre–post data can provide comparison data on the effectiveness of different teachers. ARS also provides a tool that can aid in discovering and correcting concepts not concisely communicated or perhaps miscommunicated. This "unlearning" aspect of the system helps to optimize information transfer.

## Strategies for writing good audience response questions

One good strategy for using ARS questions is to write several pretest and posttest questions for each section or for the presentation as a whole. Following are some guidelines for writing questions:

- Questions should focus on key learning objectives, not obscure trivia.
- Questions should not be too easy; a level of difficulty is necessary to inspire learners to pay attention.
- Avoid the use of trick questions to increase the difficulty.
- Avoid true/false questions, which allow guessing and remove room for improvement and evaluation of learning; if true/false questions must be used, consider also adding a "not sure" option.
- Avoid promotional-sounding statements; the audience members will know they are supposed to agree and will feel coerced or manipulated, potentially reducing the level of esteem the audience has for the instructor and for the information presented.
- Focus questions on just one element, topic, or key message so that audiences know which item is being called into question.
- Avoid fill-in-the-blank questions, which are difficult to read aloud. Keep answers separate and distinct from the question to allow for easy reading. For example, use formats such as, "Which of the following is true?" or "Which dose is recommended?"

Some examples of audience response questions are given in Table 1-5.

## Section summary: questions for audience feedback

Properly designed audience response questions can increase learning, generate interactivity, and measure progress. Audience response questions can also provide the instructor with an opportunity to clarify areas of confusion and enhance effectiveness (see Stahl and Davis, 2009c).

**TABLE 1-5:** Writing and optimizing audience response questions

| Before | Problems/Solutions | After |
|---|---|---|
| The metabolism of this drug is _____ of the cytochrome system, making the potential for cytochrome-mediated drug-drug interactions _____.<br>A. Dependent, high<br>B. Independent, low<br>C. Dependent, low<br>D. Independent, high | **Problems**<br>▶ Too many elements (focus on just one)<br>▶ Fill-in-the-blank is difficult to read aloud<br><br>**Solutions**<br>▶ Rewrite as two questions<br>▶ Rewrite with questions and answers separated (not fill-in-the-blank) | Which system is responsible for the metabolism of the drug?<br>A. Cytochromes<br>B. Glucuronidases<br>C. Oxidases<br>D. None (drug is not metabolized)<br>Cytochrome metabolism of drugs can lead to which of the following?<br>A. Poor absorption<br>B. Drug-drug interactions<br>C. Weight gain |
| Patients taking 500 mg of the drug showed an improvement in symptoms of anxiety with a good tolerability profile.<br>A. True<br>B. False | **Problems**<br>▶ Statement sounds promotional<br>▶ True/false allows for guessing<br>▶ Not clear which element (if any) is in question<br><br>**Solutions**<br>▶ Set just one element apart (dosing or disorder)<br>▶ Change from true/false format | Patients taking which dosage of the drug showed an improvement in symptoms of anxiety with a good tolerability profile?<br>A. 50 mg<br>B. 150 mg<br>C. 500 mg<br>Patients taking 500 mg of the drug experienced a good tolerability profile with an improvement in symptoms of which disorder?<br>A. Anxiety<br>B. Depression<br>C. Insomnia |

## Section 8

### Team and tandem teaching

An easy way to enliven presentations is for the main instructors to invite a guest instructor or a second instructor to join them. The change in instructors aids in accommodating audience attention span by providing additional stimulation.

Moreover, seeing the rapport between the two instructors can encourage interaction from the audience. A learning environment with two instructors feels more like a conversation and less like a lecture, so audience members feel more welcome to join – more like a part of the event than an observer. This can be especially effective when the visual materials of the presentation are not strong. Two instructors can provide a dynamic exchange of different perspectives on various issues, especially complex issues of judgment rather than straightforward interpretation of narrowly defined data.

In team teaching, in which instructors share the same presentation, instructors can develop a plan so that each one is aware of which points he or she is responsible for presenting. An alternating approach is most often advised, with planned transition points at which instructors hand off to each other. Faculty should work together ahead of time to avoid verbal tennis, banter, debate, or one-upmanship. When not presenting, instructors can position themselves less prominently than the current instructor and each instructor will want to make no more than one comment on another team member's points. The most effective arrangement in accommodating the team approach is the media style, or mutual interview, in which the instructors take on alternating roles as interviewer and interviewee.

Tandem teaching involves splitting a learning event into separate presentations or dividing sections of a presentation between instructors. The instructors decide who will deliver which lectures while making sure each is well versed in the other's material to avoid overlaps and gaps. Depending on the order of instructors, the first one will be able to preview what the following instructor will cover, while the second instructor can refer back to previous information presented by the first instructor. Each instructor will want to be able to refer ahead and back to their own or the other instructor's material. If presentations are completely separated, each instructor can remain in the room for the other presentation(s) to signal to both the audience and to the teammate that the other talk is interesting and valuable.

### Section summary: team and tandem teaching
A second instructor can make educational events more engaging for the audience and can help accommodate attention spans.

## Section 9

### Higher-impact learning formats

> *I hear and I forget.*
> *I see and I remember.*
> *I do and I understand.*                  – Chinese proverb

Different learning modalities have different retention rates, as illustrated in Figure 1-10, adapted here as the "ladder of learning" (Dale, 1969). The lowest rungs on the ladder are the most commonly used modalities, namely, self-directed learning by reading and lectures, with or without audiovisual aids. The abysmal

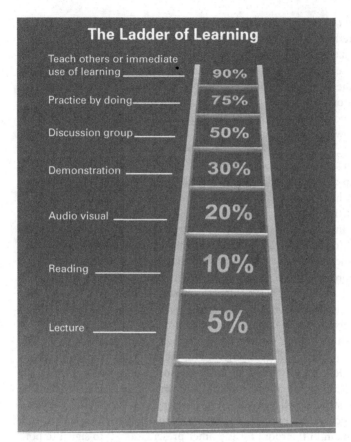

**The Ladder of Learning**

Teach others or immediate use of learning _____ 90%

Practice by doing_____ 75%

Discussion group_____ 50%

Demonstration _____ 30%

Audio visual _____ 20%

Reading _____ 10%

Lecture _____ 5%

Figure 1-10. **The ladder of learning.** (based on Dale, 1969)

retention rates of information gathered by reading are shown in many studies, including one famous analysis in which more than 3,600 subjects were instructed to read a textbook passage and were then administered a quiz at various intervals thereafter to measure retention (Spitzer, 1939). Comprehension scores were already poor on the first day and declined sharply in the days and weeks thereafter (gray trace, Figure 1-11). After 9 weeks, retention was less than 20% of original learning (black trace, Figure 1-11). Others have estimated retention rates at 72 hours after reading to be as low as 5% (Brookfield, 1986).

Listening to a lecture may be a slightly better learning format than reading alone (Figure 1-11). For example, one study of fourth-year medical students who received one-hour PowerPoint-mediated lectures once a week for 12 weeks in orthopedics showed scores on quizzes at the end of the semester that were fairly good – about 80% correct (Costa *et al.*, 2007). By contrast, when a group of the students' peers was randomized to discussion groups instead of passive lecture formats, the students in the discussion groups liked the format more and scored better on exams at the end of

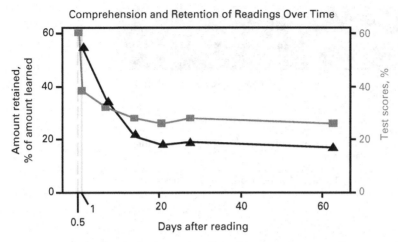

Figure 1-11. **Comprehension and retention of readings over time.** More than 3,600 subjects were given textbook passages to read and then quizzed at various intervals thereafter to measure comprehension and retention. Comprehension was based on test scores (gray trace) and was poor on the first day, declining sharply thereafter. After 9 weeks, retention (black trace) was calculated at less than 20% of original learning. (Spitzer, 1939)

the series (Costa *et al.*, 2007). This is consistent with other studies in which retention rates following a lecture approximated 10–20%, but retention rates after demonstrations were notably higher, around 30% (Figure 1-11).

Experts attribute higher retention rates on the highest rungs of the ladder to learning modalities that incorporate repetition, interactivity, multimodality, and practical application (Figure 1-10). Passive verbal receiving, found at the bottom of the ladder, or visual plus passive verbal receiving, cannot rival active forms of learning, especially doing, which also tends to have a lower degree of abstraction compared to passive reading and listening (Dale, 1969).

## Section summary: higher-impact learning formats
Educational formats that are more active and less passive can often have higher impact on learning and retention.

# Section 10

## Designing and facilitating workshops

Workshops are especially effective learning environments because they allow "discovery learning" – that is, learning in which audience members arrive at the answers themselves instead of receiving spoon-fed information from the instructor. This tactic is especially useful for medical audiences, in which learners may tend to be argumentative. One suggested "law" of adult learning is that "people do not argue with their own data" (Pike, 2008) (Table 1-6).

**TABLE 1-6**: Pike's Laws of Adult Learning

**Law 1.** Adults are babies with big bodies (so like babies, they learn by experience).

**Law 2.** People do not argue with their own data.

**Law 3.** Learning is directly proportional to the amount of fun you are having.

**Law 4.** Learning has not taken place until behavior has changed. (Pike, 1989)

If workshops or discussion groups are part of an educational event, the instructor or faculty member will be acting as a facilitator instead of a lecturer.

Following are steps to setting up and conducting a successful workshop event.

When workshops are utilized for large audiences, learners are best divided into table groups or break-out clusters. Optimum group size is five to seven people.

Workshop sections can be formed using portions of a presentation (printed and distributed slides), passages of a chapter, selections from a journal article, or different journal articles. Each table can be instructed to examine their materials and summarize them for the entire audience via the group spokesperson. The facilitator provides specific and detailed instructions appropriate to the amount of time for the workshop – for example, by asking each group to summarize each paragraph of a journal article into two key bullet points.

Instructions for the discussion time can be presented up front so all participants are aware of the format, goals, time limits, etc. Clear, concise directions given before an activity are important to obtain the desired outcomes.

A general structure for an effective workshop is given in Figure 1-12.

Once the workshop groups are formed, each group will need to appoint a spokesperson or scribe. Sometimes, designating a spokesperson can be an arduous task, and it is advised that the facilitator remain neutral and not directly make these decisions. One useful tactic is for the facilitator to ask everyone to raise a hand and point to the ceiling. When the facilitator says "go," the participants should point to the person at their table that they want as their group's spokesperson.

During the discussion time, the facilitator can walk around the room and visit each table to monitor progress. The facilitator can also help in tracking time for the groups. For example, the facilitator may announce, "We have 15 minutes left" or "One minute remaining; let's finish up." If appropriate, materials can be matched to timing. For example, five worksheets could be allotted 10 minutes each; at the

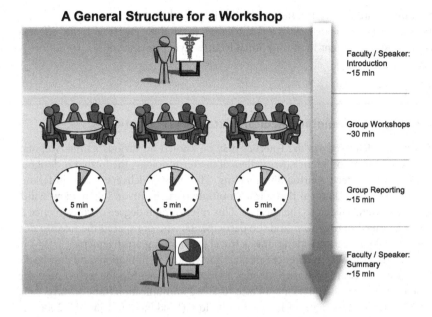

Figure 1-12. **General structure and format for an effective workshop.**

appropriate time, the instructor could announce, "Ten minutes remaining – you should be on the last worksheet by now."

Toward the end of the group discussion period, spokespersons should be reminded that they have an allotted amount of time – for example, five minutes – to present their table's results. The facilitator can then take a few minutes to compare each spokesperson's instructional knowledge with those of each group's contributions, while always complimenting each team on its answers. The facilitator can also thank each team for participating and praise the team's performance. Obviously, at the close of the session, the facilitator can summarize key learning points – both from the facilitator's own instructional materials and from the outcomes of the discussion groups – to validate each group's experience and the importance of each group's participation.

Beyond simple summarization, a first-rate facilitator will ask learners to:

- **Critique**. The learners should discuss the strengths and weaknesses of the material they are examining. The facilitator will provide clear instructions, such as, "Discuss strengths and weaknesses and select one of each to report to the group."
- **Contribute their experiences**. Medical learners bring a wealth of knowledge to the workshop. The facilitator can ask the learners to discuss the material and then discuss patients they have treated or information they have learned that is illustrative of or relevant to the material. The facilitator will want to give detailed instructions about the amount of report-back that is desired.

Section summary: designing and facilitating workshops
Workshops, when well designed and well facilitated, create a more effective learning environment than traditional lecture-style presentations.

## Section 11

### Utilizing the Internet for medical education presentations

A seminar delivered via the Internet may be known by various names: webinar, webex, and web conference. Regardless of the terminology, the format is designed to provide, in effect, a virtual live meeting. The speaker delivers a web conference using a software platform that allows multiple participants to log in, view a slide deck, and watch/listen to the speaker. This offers a high degree of convenience to both the meeting organizer and the participants, who are spared the need to deal with such logistical considerations as travel and lodging arrangements.

Of course, the web conference format is not without its limitations and drawbacks. Even if the software platform provides a video component to the web conference, much of the richness and nuance of face-to-face communication (tone of voice, facial expressions, body language) is likely to be lost (Häkkinen and Järvelä, 2006). In addition, because web conferencing relies so heavily on networking technology, there is an inherent risk that technical difficulties (e.g. slow streaming speeds, network disconnections) may negatively impact the learning experience.

The potential for a webinar to provide an effective, collaborative learning environment rests as much in the capabilities of the platform as in the presenting capabilities of the speaker. For example, some webinar formats allow question-and-answer sessions and audience polling. These interactive features allow for a maximization of learner participation and should therefore be included whenever possible. It is also very helpful to provide slides notes to the participants in advance to facilitate optimal learning.

In summary, here are some factors that you should consider in planning your web conference (Archer, 2004):

- *Web conference provider.* Who will provide the platform for your web conference? The answer to this question will depend on the participation volume you expect (both number of web conferences and number of participants). Prices are usually lowest for higher volume. Availability of support services may vary, but in general will be greater for high-end price options.
- *Platform technology.* The capabilities of the platform will dictate what you can do with your presentation. For example, Java and Flash offer different feature sets that may affect how your program is executed.
- *Presentation features.* In addition to the audience polling that has already been mentioned, other features of web conferences may enhance the learning experience of participants. These features include: pointer and annotation tools; chat (allowing two-way communication between the meeting presenter and participants); multiple presenters; and a dynamic "white board" interface that permits

information sharing. In general, dynamic features allow the greatest degree of collaboration and interactivity, and are the most expensive and difficult to use.

● *Audio.* Some web conference platforms may deliver only the visual component (namely, the slide deck), with the audio component provided by a parallel conference call that requires separate "dial-in" by all participants. In this case, it is advisable to provide operator assistance, to alleviate management burden from the presenter.

### Section summary: utilizing the Internet for medical education presentations

Webinars are seminars or presentations delivered over the Internet, allowing for a convenient and wide-reaching delivery of medical education. They can be very effective when they include audience preparation and participation.

## Chapter summary

● Slide enhancements that meet the needs of adult education principles can include preview and review sections, visual translations, and small multiples.

● The principles of multimedia learning (modality, contiguity, coherence, and redundancy) should be taken into account during design of individual slides to increase the potential for key messages to reach the target audience.

● Theories such as the "events of instruction" and the "conditions of learning" can help instructors evaluate the design of presentations and educational programs and develop a plan for how best to convey education materials to a medical audience.

● The use of audience response system questions can dramatically increase educational impact and audience engagement.

● A second instructor can enliven instructional events and play to the attention spans of an audience.

● Designing and facilitating a workshop, instead of giving a didactic lecture, can engage learners and increase their knowledge retention.

## Progress check

Write down your answers in the pages provided in the back of the book or on a separate piece of paper so that you can retake this test periodically without bias from your previous markings. Check your answers against the key in the back of the book and record your score in the ledger at the end of this quiz.

1. With one exception, all of the following are useful for parceling out your information into small multiples. Which does not belong?
   a. Similarities and differences
   b. Before and after

      c. Parallel structure

      d. Preview and review

2. Which of the following is not a helpful visual addition?

      a. Three-dimensional effects on charts

      b. Converting a table to a bar chart

      c. Converting statistics to a pie chart

      d. Anatomical photographs or figures

3. The modality principle of multimedia learning suggests that learners benefit from learning information

      a. Auditorily and textually

      b. Auditorily and visually

      c. Visually and textually

      d. Visually, textually, and auditorily

4. The redundancy principle of multimedia learning suggests that learners may be

      a. Bored by repetition of concepts

      b. Distracted by extraneous on-screen text

      c. Put off by repeated adjectives, such as "very, very large"

5. The contiguity principle of multimedia learning states that

      a. Information should flow like a continuous story plot line

      b. Learning is facilitated when related information is paired spatially

      c. Learning is facilitated when related information is paired temporally

      d. Both b and c

6. According to the "events of instruction," three of the following must happen before an instructor can present new information. Which does not belong? The instructor must:

      a. Gain and control attention

      b. Describe expected outcomes

      c. Offer guidance for learning

      d. Refer to previous learning

7. Three of the following are "conditions of learning" for adults. Which does not belong?

      a. Involvement – learners must be psychologically invested in learning

      b. Challenge – previous learning must be called into question

      c. Discipline – learners must trust that the instructor will maintain order in the audience

      d. Support – learners need an open and empathetic environment

8. Which of the following is a good question for giving feedback to gauge audience understanding?

      a. A true/false question

      b. A multiple choice question

      c. A fill-in-the-blank question

9. According to the principles suggested in the "ladder of learning," which type of instruction is likely to have the highest impact?

      a. Participating in a discussion group

      b. Reading a textbook that contains images

      c. Hearing an audio broadcast

      d. Watching a presentation that contains images

## Performance ledger

| Assessment | Date | Scoring |
|---|---|---|
| 1 | | # correct answers:<br>percent correct answers (divide by 9): |
| 2 | | # correct answers:<br>percent correct answers (divide by 9): |
| 3 | | # correct answers:<br>percent correct answers (divide by 9): |
| 4 | | # correct answers:<br>percent correct answers (divide by 9): |
| 5 | | # correct answers:<br>percent correct answers (divide by 9): |

## Performance self-assessment

Photocopy this page or write down your answers on a separate piece of paper so that you can retake this assessment periodically without bias from your previous markings. Record your score in the ledger on the next page.

| | 1 | 2 | 3 | 4 | 5 |
|---|---|---|---|---|---|
| | Poor, or Strongly Disagree | Fair, or Disagree | Average, or Neutral | Good, or Agree | Great, or Strongly Agree |
| **Slide deck structure** | | | | | |
| **1.** My slide decks contain initial and recurrent outline slides to give previews to the audiences. | ☐ | ☐ | ☐ | ☐ | ☐ |
| **2.** Each section of my slide deck contains a review and summary slide. | ☐ | ☐ | ☐ | ☐ | ☐ |
| **3.** I plan activities to gain and control attention at the beginning of an instructional event. | ☐ | ☐ | ☐ | ☐ | ☐ |

| | 1 | 2 | 3 | 4 | 5 |
|---|---|---|---|---|---|
| 4. I refer to previous learning before presenting new information. | ☐ | ☐ | ☐ | ☐ | ☐ |
| 5. I pose structured questions to the audience for feedback that allows them to gauge their performance. | ☐ | ☐ | ☐ | ☐ | ☐ |
| **Individual slides** | | | | | |
| 6. I add helpful visual elements – charts, figures, images – wherever appropriate. | ☐ | ☐ | ☐ | ☐ | ☐ |
| 7. I eliminate extraneous on-screen text. | ☐ | ☐ | ☐ | ☐ | ☐ |
| 8. I parcel text and images into small multiples. | ☐ | ☐ | ☐ | ☐ | ☐ |
| 9. I make my data visually contiguous. | ☐ | ☐ | ☐ | ☐ | ☐ |
| 10. I eliminate information that is only padding or tangential to the main points. | ☐ | ☐ | ☐ | ☐ | ☐ |
| **Alternative formats** | | | | | |
| 11. I have worked successfully with a second presenter. | ☐ | ☐ | ☐ | ☐ | ☐ |
| 12. I have successfully designed and facilitated a workshop. | ☐ | ☐ | ☐ | ☐ | ☐ |
| Total number of checkmarks per column: | – | – | – | – | – |

## Performance self-assessment score sheet

| | | | 1 | 2 | 3 | 4 | 5 |
|---|---|---|---|---|---|---|---|
| Assessment | Date | Scoring | | | | | |
| Sample | 23 July 2009 | # items with each score: | $1 \times 1$ | $3 \times 2$ | $3 \times 3$ | $3 \times 4$ | $2 \times 5$ |
| | | Value | 1 | 6 | 9 | 12 | 10 |
| | | Total score (sum of value line): 38 | | | | | |
| | | Percent success (divide score by maximum, 60): 63% | | | | | |
| 1 | | # items with each score: | $\times 1$ | $\times 2$ | $\times 3$ | $\times 4$ | $\times 5$ |
| | | Value | | | | | |
| | | Total score (sum of value line): | | | | | |
| | | Percent success (divide score by maximum, 55): | | | | | |

| Assessment | Date | Scoring | | | | | |
|---|---|---|---|---|---|---|---|
| 2 | | # items with each score: | ×1 | ×2 | ×3 | ×4 | ×5 |
| | | Value | | | | | |
| | | Total score (sum of value line): | | | | | |
| | | Percent success (divide score by maximum, 55): | | | | | |
| 3 | | # items with each score: | ×1 | ×2 | ×3 | ×4 | ×5 |
| | | Value | | | | | |
| | | Total score (sum of value line): | | | | | |
| | | Percent success (divide score by maximum, 55): | | | | | |
| 4 | | # items with each score: | ×1 | ×2 | ×3 | ×4 | ×5 |
| | | Value | | | | | |
| | | Total score (sum of value line): | | | | | |
| | | Percent success (divide score by maximum, 55): | | | | | |
| 5 | | # items with each score: | ×1 | ×2 | ×3 | ×4 | ×5 |
| | | Value | | | | | |
| | | Total score (sum of value line): | | | | | |
| | | Percent success (divide score by maximum, 55): | | | | | |

# Using audience learning psychology to advantage in designing and delivering medical presentations

## Chapter overview

Chapter 2 examines those characteristics that all audiences have in common, starting from the moment just before people walk into the meeting room. Emphasis is given

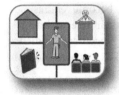

to the characteristics that are most common in members of a medical audience.

The first section explains how to settle **tensions in the learning environment**. Audiences experience four tensions that have the potential to distract at least some of them from an instructor's message: discomfort in the room, tensions with the other learners, unfamiliarity with the instructor, and tension with the material and the process of the presentation. Instructors who are aware of these tensions can relieve them, thereby making audiences more receptive to instruction.

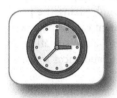

Even after audience members settle down, they will be able to pay attention only for a limited amount of time. The next section will discuss ways to accommodate **the attention span of audience members** to ensure they are highly interested and fully focused throughout a presentation.

Each audience member's receptiveness to a presentation, or to any given part of a presentation, depends in part on his or her learning style. Understanding and accommodating the **four learning styles** – visual, auditory, reading/writing, and kinesthetic/tactile – can help an instructor develop and implement a presentation that is more effective for a greater portion of the audience.

Different learners will want to use newly acquired information in different ways – either for problem solving (convergent thinking) or for idea generating (divergent

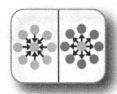

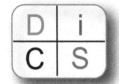

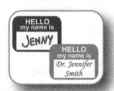

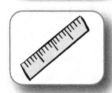

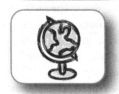

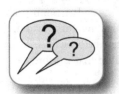

thinking). Accommodating **the two thinking styles** can increase the proportion of audience members who are receptive to a presentation.

An instructor can also reach more learners and educate them more thoroughly by knowing about different personality styles and understanding what a person with each different style seeks from a learning experience. One way among many to classify **personality types** of audience members is the DiSC profile, which characterizes audience members by the traits of dominance, influence, steadiness, and conscientiousness.

Adult medical audiences have a wealth of relevant experience. Drawing on this experience can add impact to an instructor's presentation. Conversely, neglecting it can reduce an audience's receptiveness. This section explains how to use **audience experience** to improve a presentation.

Adult medical learners are most motivated to learn when they self-diagnose a need for knowledge. By helping audience members measure their present level of understanding and discover their own need for learning, an instructor can inspire them to become enthusiastic about (instead of just resigned to) their role as learners. This section demonstrates how to encourage **audience self-assessment** during a presentation as a way to motivate attendees to learn.

Adult medical learners are less interested in abstract knowledge, trivia, or bits of arcana than they are in useful information – tools they can use. Emphasizing the **practical application** of instructional content can help audiences imagine using information from a presentation in everyday situations. This will motivate audiences to listen, learn, and remember.

Medical audiences often contain learners from a variety of cultures; these learners, in turn, may provide health care to patients of varying ethnicities. Data can be translated and behavior modified to accommodate this **cultural diversity**. By adopting a wider world view, an instructor can draw more learners in and make content more meaningful to a global audience.

Medical audiences include eager and sometimes combative questioners. The last section will cover how to **respond to audience questions** appropriately in order to appear knowledgeable and helpful while enhancing learning for the entire audience.

# Introduction

## Rationale and benefits

In order to learn, audience members must first be comfortable and ready to participate in the educational process. A secure environment with few distractions will make an audience optimally receptive to an instructor's message.

Members of all audiences – even physicians – have a limited attention span. In addition, different audience members have different learning styles and personality characteristics that influence learning. All of these factors – attention span, learning styles, and personality traits – can be accommodated to increase an instructor's educational effectiveness.

In addition to possessing the characteristics of ordinary audiences, medical learners are a mature, sophisticated group. In order to help these audience members achieve their learning goals, it is quite useful for an instructor to understand their unique perspective. This will allow the instructor to lead audience members to greater self-awareness and mastery of the content being presented.

This chapter shows how paying attention to the characteristics of learners can help a medical educator succeed in effectively conveying knowledge and enhancing his or her image as a competent instructor.

# Section 1

## Tensions in the learning environment

When learners enter the room where they will be receiving instruction, they experience four tensions that can inhibit their learning: environmental tension, tension with other learners, learner–instructor tension, and tension stemming from the material and process to be used. An unaware instructor might try to talk over the top of these tensions, but until these issues are addressed, learners are not listening – they have not yet reached their "receptive point," as shown in Figure 2-1.

### Environmental tension
Especially on their first visit to a learning venue, learners will experience tension stemming from the environment. Even familiar locations can include discomforting elements that require an instructor's continued attention and maintenance. Although many times it is not possible, arriving early at the venue – especially for presentations to a large audience – allows an instructor the chance to minimize the potential for learner tensions before any participants arrive, as shown in Table 2-1. It is essential to ensure that everyone can see the instructor and the presentation, that the room temperature is comfortable, and that there is ample room for note taking. Final steps for removing environmental tensions include requesting that cell phones be turned off and pointing out the locations of facilities (lavatories, vending machines, drinking fountains, etc.).

> **TABLE 2-1:** Checklist for minimizing environmental tensions during room setup
>
> ✓ Walk around the room. Familiarize yourself with the space and note how it feels in different locations. Check for sight lines and glare.
>
> ✓ Learn the lighting controls (both windows and switches). Ideal lighting will keep your audience awake but will also allow high-contrast projection of your slides.
>
> ✓ Check the room temperature. Where are the controls? How will the temperature change when the room is filled?
>
> ✓ Ensure that learners have space to spread out (and write on) their educational materials.
>
> ✓ Become familiar with the proper operation of any audiovisual equipment being used (e.g., slide advance remote).
>
> (Vosko, 1991)

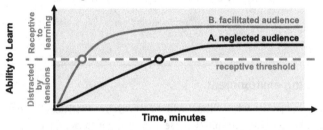

Figure 2-1. **Settling tensions to reach the receptive point.** Using preparation and introduction time to address learner tensions will bring audience members to their "receptive point" sooner. In a neglected audience scenario (dark gray trace), the instructor launches immediately into lecturing without addressing the tensions of the learners. The audience members eventually reach a receptive point (dashed line) after they settle some of their tensions by looking around the room or by using effort to ignore those tensions. In a facilitated audience scenario (light gray trace), the instructor is aware of the tensions in the audience and takes a few minutes of introduction to address these needs. Compared to the neglected audience, the facilitated audience reaches the receptive point (dashed line) much sooner, which increases participants' overall ability to learn.

## Learner-to-learner tension

Although not usually done for formal lecture settings, for instructors who wish to utilize discussion groups and workshops, it is useful to build an environment that will encourage interaction and minimize tension among learners. Most classical lectures utilize "sociofugal" seating, which focuses on one person (the instructor)

## Seating Arrangements to Foster Learner Interactions

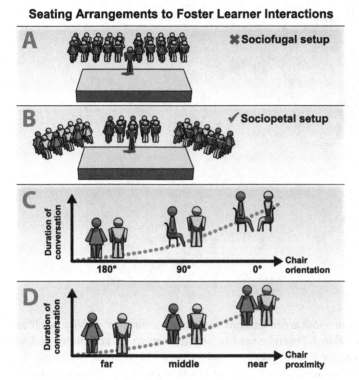

Figure 2-2. **Seating arrangements to foster learner interactions.** Sociofugal setups (A) discourage interactions among participants, whereas sociopetal environments (B) invite interactions. Chair orientation (C) can also affect interactivity: a side-by-side arrangement facilitates the least interaction; a face-to-face setup encourages the most conversation. Chair proximity (D) also affects interactivity: learners talk most when they are closer together. Therefore, as the audience fills the room, attendees of a workshop or discussion group should be discouraged from sitting too far away from one another. (Mehrabian and Diamond, 1971)

and by design invites no interaction among participants (Figure 2-2A). The suffix fugal comes from a Latin word meaning "to put to flight"; thus, sociofugal seating makes participants feel detached from each other and linked only to the speaker.

For discussion groups and workshops, "sociopetal" seating is preferred, which allows participation in the learning activity and encourages interaction among learners (Figure 2-2B). The suffix petal comes from a Latin word meaning "to seek"; thus, sociopetal seating makes participants feel more connected to each other. In short, instructors can set the learners up, depending upon the format of the presentation. These contrasting seating arrangements have been studied in classical psychology experiments by Alfred Mehrabian (Mehrabian and Diamond, 1971; see Figure 2-2 and BioBox 2-1).

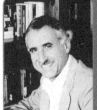

**BIOBOX 2-1**

**Albert Mehrabian**

▸ Born 1939

▸ BS and MS in engineering from Massachusetts Institute of Technology

▸ PhD in psychology from Clark University

▸ At press time for this book, was Professor Emeritus of Psychology at the University of California, Los Angeles

▸ Studied and published extensively on
  – nonverbal communication, especially body language
  – the psychology of names
  – the psychology of environments and surroundings
  – rating scales for measuring emotion

To reduce learner-to-learner tensions further, an icebreaker activity (such as those shown in Table 2-2) can be used to help learners to get acquainted and to realize that they share similar questions and feelings. This tactic is not frequently used in formal medical lecture settings but can be useful if the group is going to interact over time, such as in a class of students, or even over a series of hours or days, such as in a symposium or course.

### Learner–instructor tension

When meeting an instructor for the first time, learners will experience tension due to their unfamiliarity with the new instructor. However, audience members can be made to feel more comfortable with their instructor at the beginning and throughout a presentation. Prior to the beginning of the meeting, the instructor can move through the room and meet as many people as time will allow. This effort can help an instructor to start building audience rapport even before the meeting actually starts.

During the introduction, the instructor can establish credibility and authenticity with learners by indicating his or her qualifications or by telling something about himself or herself. The instructor can also describe any education and experience that is relevant to the material in the presentation or that may be similar to that of the audience. The instructor can clarify whether he or she will be open to questions and whether questions may be asked throughout the presentation or at a designated period at the end of the event.

### Learner–material tension

Of course, most audience members will be unfamiliar with the new material being presented. Familiarizing them with the content is the purpose of the instruction,

**TABLE 2-2:** Icebreaker activities to reduce tension between learners

**Introductions:**  Each person gives his or her name and some relevant piece of background that the leader specifies (reason for attending the presentation, college attended, specialty of practice). Depending on the size of the audience, attendees can do this in pairs, in groups, or with the whole room.

---

**Name Chain:** Participants introduce themselves, giving a name and one word of self-description. Each person in the chain repeats all previous names and descriptors. The leader is the final link in the chain, giving the list with the name of each attendee. The leader's own descriptive word can be relevant to the instructional topic, such as college attended or medical specialty: "Psychiatrist Dave, Rheumatologist Li, Endocrinologist Nancy" or "Arizona Amy, Stanford Sue, Harvard Henry."

---

**Finding Commonalities:**  If the audience is a small group or if it can be divided into table groups, participants can be asked to find something they have in common among themselves. Examples include hair color, shoe size, or a movie everyone has seen—or, the commonality might be more relevant to the educational topic, such as common memberships in a professional society or subscriptions to a journal.

---

(Sisco, 1991)

but the instructor will not want to dive into the material until the other three tensions have been addressed. Once the other three tensions have been attended to, the instructor can summarize the material to come (both objectives and content). The instructor can also introduce any accompanying printed materials. This may involve explaining that there is a handout or letting learners know how to get a handout later. The instructor can also let learners know that the handout will provide a presentation overview or agenda and information on how questions will be handled.

## Section summary: tensions in the learning environment

Learners experience four tensions: environmental tension, learner-to-learner tension, learner–instructor tension, and learner–material tension. If these tensions are relieved during presentation setup and introduction, learners will reach their receptive point more quickly, and they will be able to give more attention to the presentation.

## Section 2

### The attention span of audiences

For learners who are not distracted by the four tensions, attention will be at a maximum at the beginning of a presentation. It will quickly begin to fall away, as shown in Figure 2-3 (dashed trace). Adult learners can stay tuned in to a lecture for no more than 15 to 20 minutes at a time, and that is only at the beginning of the presentation. As presentations proceed, lapses in learner attention come more frequently. The second lapse occurs after about 10 to 18 minutes, and by the end of a lecture, attention span is only three to four minutes (Middendorf and Kalish, 1996).

Attention span may also be dependent on the time of day and the hunger level of the listeners. Therefore, when the presentation is longer than 20 minutes, the instructor needs to do something to accommodate the attention span of the audience, as shown in Figure 2-3 (black trace). Otherwise, after that time, many in the audience will be tuning out and drifting away as they lose their ability to pay attention.

Change-ups are periodic activities that can be used to accommodate attention span. A sampler of change-ups is given in Table 2-3. One extremely effective change-up is the section review. This tactic involves finding the natural breaks in presentation material to divide it into smaller topics. Change-ups can be facilitated by asking questions at key points throughout the lecture and by utilizing audience response keypads, a tactic that will be discussed in detail later in this book.

Although rarely used in medical presentations due to the press of time, at the end of each section the instructor can consider allowing small groups in the

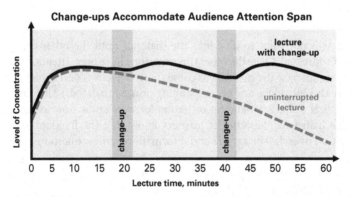

Figure 2-3. **Change-ups accommodate audience attention span.** As a presentation proceeds, learners lose their ability to concentrate. The dashed trace shows the approximate extrapolated concentration levels in a medical presentation audience. Adding change-ups to a presentation, as shown in the black trace, can accommodate the attention span of audience members. (Stuart and Rutherford, 1978)

**TABLE 2-3**: Change-ups to accommodate learner attention span

**Questions**

- ▸ The instructor can ask questions about key points of content in a section.

- ▸ The instructor can take audience questions during a change-up.

- ▸ The instructor can ask all learners to write down one to three questions that arose during the preceding section of a presentation and then take verbal questions from volunteers.

- ▸ The instructor can ask learners to write exam questions based on the material that was just presented.

**Reviews**

- ▸ Participants can summarize material in discussion groups.

- ▸ The instructor can give the reviews if discussion groups are impractical.

**Controversial topics**

- ▸ After presenting a controversial topic, the instructor can ask learners to answer questions such as, "Which ideas do you question?" or "What ideas are new to you?" Discussion on the topic can take place in small groups or can involve the entire audience.

- ▸ Learners can move to a place that represents their feelings about a topic. For example, assenters can move to the right side of the room while dissenters move to the left side. One learner from each group can be paired with a learner from the opposite group to generate a debate. One option is for debaters to argue for the opposing side to allow them to understand a viewpoint that is different from their own.

**Media variations**

- ▸ If learner participation events are impractical, change-ups can be built into a presentation with different media types. For example, an instructor can use a video clip (such as a case study) or a sound file (such as an audio recording of a functioning organ or a patient self-report of symptoms).

(Middendorf and Kalish, 1996)

audience (table groups or paired partners) to discuss two or three key takeaway points from the preceding section of the presentation. To close the break, the leader can call on each group to report back its findings. If it is impractical to allow discussion, the instructor can give the reviews. Section reviews allow listeners to package away each set of information and then turn to a new topic with fresh interest.

Other tactics include showing joke slides or telling a humorous anecdote. And a serious case example to close out a section or introduce another section generally changes the pace of the presentation and can recapture the attention of the audience. Another tactic is for the instructor to ask questions of the audience about the information that was just presented. Use of a variety of techniques, depending on the length of the presentation, can raise the level of sustained audience engagement.

### Section summary: the attention span of audiences

Audiences have an attention span that starts short and gets shorter as the presentation continues. Change-ups in a presentation can keep audience attention at a maximum.

## Section 3

### The four learning styles

An instructor giving a presentation in a traditional format might do everything "right" but still leave some learners behind. One reason for this disparity is that not everyone learns well from a live lecture presentation format. Different people learn in different ways. Moreover, each instructor is prone to present in his or her own learning style, which will not match every learner in the audience. In fact, audience members can typically be characterized as being one of four learner types:

1. visual types
2. auditory types
3. reading/writing types
4. kinesthetic/tactile types.

### The four learner types in a medical audience

Various learning styles can be accommodated during a presentation. In fact, most medical learners (~64%) prefer educational formats that incorporate a variety of styles; that is, most are "multimodal" learners. One study of first-year medical students in the USA found the distribution of learner types shown in Figure 2-4. Another study of 155 first-year medical students in Turkey found a similar distribution: 64% multimodal, 23% kinesthetic, 8% auditory, 3% visual, and 2% reading/writing (Baykan and Nacar, 2007).

### Visual learners

Of the multimodal learners in the two studies mentioned, most (75% in the US study, 55% in the Turkish study) prefer learning that includes a visual element, so it

**The Four Learner Types in a Medical Audience**

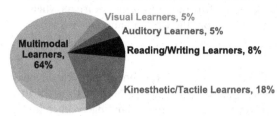

Figure 2-4. **The four learner types in a medical audience.** This distribution is from a study of 166 first-year medical students (Lujan and DiCarlo, 2006); the distribution in other audiences may vary.

may be especially important to accommodate visual learners. Visual types learn best through seeing drawings, pictures, and other image-rich instructional tools. Visual learners or visual-multimodal learners will focus on the illustrative elements of a presentation, such as diagrams, symbols, graphs, flow charts, hierarchies, figures, and models. Therefore, adding visual elements to a presentation will aid these learners. During a presentation, visual learners or visual-multimodal learners might benefit from taking color-coded or highlighted notes or including sketches of graphs or figures; educational impact will be increased if these learners are given the space and resources (colored pencils, paper, etc.) to add visuals to their notes.

## Auditory learners

Auditory types learn best by listening to lectures, by exploring material through discussions, and by talking about ideas. Auditory learners or auditory-multimodal learners will focus on what is said during a presentation, answers given during any question-and-answer sessions, and any discussions allowed or mediated during the presentation. Auditory learners or auditory-multimodal learners may benefit from use of word associations or mnemonics, from recording the lectures for later listening, from reading their notes on the lecture out loud to themselves later, or from articulating their ideas during group discussions at a change-up. An instructor who keeps questions to a minimum, runs long, or cuts off questioning at the end can cheat this type of learner.

## Reading/writing learners

Reading/writing types learn best through interaction with text or written materials. Reading/writing learners or reading/writing-multimodal learners will focus on the statements written out on slides or on lecture notes, handouts, or textbooks that accompany the presentation. Reading/writing learners or reading/writing-multimodal learners benefit especially from translation of verbal information into written notes and from organization of information into lists or glossaries. Such learners can become quite upset and frustrated if the instructor does not follow his or her own handout, adds new slides, or changes the order of slides.

Thus, the instructor can decide whether the trade-off of flexibility of revising the lecture up to the last minute is worth the frustration to certain learners when the presentation materials vary significantly from the written handout.

### Kinesthetic/tactile learners

Kinesthetic/tactile types learn through touching, experiences, physical involvement, and manipulation of objects. These types may be hardest to reach in a traditional lecture or presentation format, and they may seem fidgety when forced to sit still for long lectures. Kinesthetic/tactile learners or kinesthetic/tactile-multimodal learners will focus on simulations of real practices and experiences in a presentation, such as case studies or role-playing. They will appreciate the opportunity to handle any tangible aids that can be passed around during a talk, such as preserved pathology slides or anatomical models. These learners benefit from being allowed to move during a learning event, such as rotating to a discussion group and then back to their lecture seats during a change-up.

### Section summary: the four learning styles

Audience members may prefer different learning modes, such as auditory, visual, reading/writing, or kinesthetic/tactile styles. By accommodating different learning styles, an instructor can reach more learners and educate them more thoroughly.

## Section 4

### The two thinking styles

In addition to the four learning styles, audience members also have two different thinking styles: convergent and divergent. Convergent thinkers focus on problem solving, and they gather information to generate answers. These thinkers flourish when taking multiple-choice tests, for which each question has a single correct answer. In fact, a lifetime of test-taking encourages convergent thinking. In contrast to convergent thinkers, divergent thinkers generate ideas from some central stimulus or fact. Instead of a single correct answer to a question, they might perceive a host of possibilities. Divergent thinkers flourish when brainstorming. A schematic depicting the thought processes of convergent and divergent thinkers is shown in Figure 2-5.

In a study of 52 surgical trainees, the majority (60%) were convergent thinkers (Drew et al., 1999). Divergent thinking among medical learners may decrease with experience or with exposure to testing. In another study of 17 pediatric residents and 22 faculty, residents tended toward divergence, but faculty tended toward convergence (Kosower and Berman, 1996). Thus, an experienced medical audience might consist mostly of convergent thinkers, but they will learn more thoroughly when encouraged to look at information from both standpoints, as shown in Table 2-4.

**TABLE 2-4**: Methods to encourage different thinking styles in learners

**Suggestions for divergent thinking**
When presenting a new idea, an instructor can ask learners to generate other ideas along the same line.

| When presenting about... | | Instructors can ask learners to name... |
|---|---|---|
| side effects of a drug | → | drugs with similar side effects |
| pathology of a disease or disorder | → | diseases or disorders with similar pathology |
| symptoms reported by certain patients | → | conditions leading to similar symptoms |

**Suggestions for convergent thinking**
When presenting a new idea, an instructor can ask learners to apply the knowledge to solve a problem.

| When presenting about... | | Instructors can ask learners to use the knowledge to name... |
|---|---|---|
| pathology of a disease or disorder | → | drugs that target the pathology |
| mode of action of a drug | → | conditions possibly treatable by the drug |
| symptoms of a condition | → | screening questions or tests for diagnosis |

## Convergent Versus Divergent Thinking

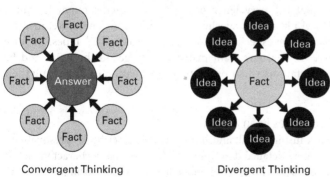

Convergent Thinking      Divergent Thinking

Figure 2-5. **Convergent versus divergent thinking.** Convergent thinkers want to gather facts to solve a problem; divergent thinkers want to use facts to generate new ideas.

### Section summary: the two thinking styles

Audience members may tend toward divergent thinking (idea generating) or convergent thinking (problem solving). By accommodating different thinking styles, an instructor can increase audience engagement with and retention of the material being presented.

## Section 5

### Personality types

An individual's personality type has a profound effect on that person's learning style. Instructors with an ongoing relationship with their learners may have time to learn their individual personalities and respond appropriately. Otherwise, simply being aware of the diversity in an audience can help an instructor speak more broadly in order to reach all types. There are a variety of ways to categorize personality types, including the Myers-Briggs type indicator (Myers *et al.*, 1998), the enneagram of personality (Riso and Hudson, 1996), and the DiSC assessment, which will be discussed here.

In the DiSC system, the personalities of most people can be described using one of four classifications. The "D" types, or dominance types, like to be in charge and are decisive about the way to do things. The "i" types, or influence types, are enthusiastic and persuasive. The "S" types, or steadiness types, are the ultimate team players, always supportive and friendly. The "C" types, or conscientiousness types, are careful and quiet.

### "D" (dominance) personalities in an audience

"D" personalities are dominant, demanding, and determined. A more detailed description of "D" personality characteristics is given in Table 2-5. The estimated prevalence of people with "D" as their strongest trait in the general public is about 10%, but surveys and small case reports of those in the medical profession suggest that the prevalence of "D"s in medicine might be much higher – up to 75% of physicians, as shown in Figure 2-6. Therefore, medical instructors may want to be especially prepared to speak to "D" types. Because of their personality, "D" learners want instructors to get to the point and be clear about their expectations when presenting information or answering their questions.

### "i" (influence) personalities in an audience

The words influencer, inspirational, and interactive all describe "i" personalities. Table 2-6 provides a more detailed description of "i" personality characteristics. It is estimated that about 30% of the general public has "i" as their strongest trait and that the rate is similar among medical professionals (Figure 2-7). Because of their personality, "i" types want the instructor to be relaxed, humorous, and sociable

**TABLE 2-5**: Characteristics of the "D" type personality

| | |
|---|---|
| "D" emphasis | Shaping the environment by overcoming opposition and challenges |
| "D" tendencies | Getting immediate results, taking action, accepting challenges, making quick decisions |
| "D" motivations | Challenges power and authority, direct answers, opportunities for individual accomplishments |
| "D" fears | Loss of control of the environment, being taken advantage of |
| Instructor will notice | Self-confidence, decisiveness, risk taking |

(InScape Publishing, 1996)

**TABLE 2-6**: Characteristics of the "i" type personality

| | |
|---|---|
| "i" emphasis | Shaping the environment by persuading and influencing others |
| "i" tendencies | Being involved with people, making a favorable impression, entertaining, participating in groups |
| "i" motivations | Social recognition, group activities, relationships, freedom of expression, freedom from control |
| "i" fears | Social rejection, disapproval, loss of influence |
| Instructor will notice | Enthusiasm, charm, sociability, persuasiveness, expression of emotion |

(InScape Publishing, 1996)

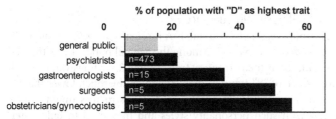

Figure 2-6. **Prevalence of the "D" type personality in selected medical professions.** Data were generated from estimates of general population (InScape Publishing, 1996) and from surveys of physicians attending speaker-training events. (Arbor Scientia, 1999, 2007, 2008)

**TABLE 2-7:** Characteristics of the "S" type personality

| | |
|---|---|
| "S" emphasis | Achieving stability, accomplishing tasks by cooperating with others |
| "S" tendencies | Calmness, patience, loyalty, good listening skills |
| "S" motivations | Minimizing change, maintaining stability, earning sincere appreciation, gaining cooperation, using traditional methods |
| "S" fears | Loss of stability, the unknown, change, unpredictability |
| Instructor will notice | Patience, stability, methodical approach, easy-going nature, concern for the group, being a team player |

(InScape Publishing, 1996)

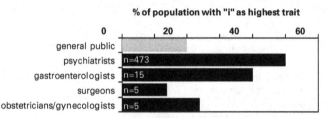

**% of population with "i" as highest trait**

Figure 2-7. **Prevalence of the "i" type personality in selected medical professions.** Data were generated from estimates of general population (InScape Publishing, 1996) and from surveys of physicians attending speaker-training events. (Arbor Scientia, 1999, 2007, 2008)

with them; when they contribute to a presentation or to a discussion, they want the leader to recognize their accomplishments.

## "S" (steadiness) personalities in an audience

"S" personalities are supportive, steady, and stable. A more specific description of "S" personality traits is provided in Table 2-7. Among the general public, the estimated prevalence of people with "S" as their strongest trait is about 35%; however, research suggests that the prevalence of "S"-types in medicine might be much lower than in the general population (Figure 2-8). Therefore, medical instructors might not be accustomed to dealing with such personality styles and may need to tailor their behaviors especially for "S" types in their audience. "S" types want the instructor to be logical and systematic and to provide a secure environment. For example, the leader can choose a volunteer only from those who are raising their hands to answer a question.

**TABLE 2-8**: Characteristics of the "C" type personality

| | |
|---|---|
| "C" emphasis | Working within circumstances to ensure quality and accuracy |
| "C" tendencies | Attention to standards and details, analytical thinking, accuracy, diplomacy, indirect approaches to conflict |
| "C" motivations | Clearly defined performance expectations, quality and accuracy, reserved and businesslike atmosphere, articulated standards |
| "C" fears | Criticism of their work, slipshod methods, situations emotionally out of control |
| Instructor will notice | Cautiousness, restraint, factuality, precision, diplomacy, perfectionism |

(InScape Publishing, 1996)

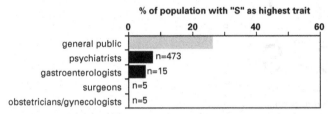

Figure 2-8. **Prevalence of the "S" type personality in selected medical professions.** Data were generated from estimates of general population (InScape Publishing, 1996) and from surveys of physicians attending speaker-training events. (Arbor Scientia, 1999, 2007, 2008)

## "C" (conscientiousness) personalities in an audience

"C" personalities are competent, cautious, and calculating. Table 2-8 offers more details about "C" type personality traits. About 25% of people have "C" as their strongest trait, but surveys reveal a wide variance in the percentage of "C" types in different medical specialties (Figure 2-9). "C" types want the instructor to be tactful and emotionally reserved when answering their questions, and they prefer to learn from instructors who use precedents as guides for new information.

## Personality-based learner focus in an audience

In addition to being aware of how an individual's personality influences the way he or she prefers to be managed, it is also helpful for an instructor to think of the group as a whole, catering in some way to each personality type, as shown in Figure 2-10. This will ensure that the message reaches a greater number of audience members.

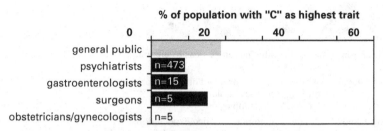

Figure 2-9. **Prevalence of the "C" type personality in selected medical professions.** Data were generated from estimates of general population (InScape Publishing, 1996) and from surveys of physicians attending speaker-training events. (Arbor Scientia, 1999, 2007, 2008)

## Focus and Pace in Learner Personalities

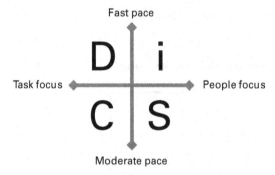

Figure 2-10. **Focus and pace in learner personalities.** Dominance and influence types prefer faster pacing, while steadiness and conscientiousness types prefer more moderate pacing. Influence and steadiness types like information that relates to people, such as their patients; dominance and conscientiousness types are more focused on tasks and problem solving, such as how to make quicker diagnoses.

Dominance ("D") and influence ("i") types prefer fast-paced learning environments. Therefore, if a discussion gets bogged down in detailed questions, the instructor might ask the questioners to meet after the learning session to prevent boring the "D"-types and "i"-types with the slower pace. Conversely, if an instructor is covering topics quickly, the instructor will want to consider giving the conscientiousness ("C") and steadiness ("S") personalities an opportunity for learning at a more deliberate pace. For example, the instructor might acknowledge that he or she is moving quickly and invite interested learners to stay after the presentation for a more in-depth discussion. As an alternative, the instructor might point learners to materials or resources that will allow them to study at their leisure.

Personality types also differ in their focus during learning. Because influence ("i") and steadiness ("S") types are focused on people, they appreciate instructors relating their information to people, such as patients or colleagues. For example, the instructor could focus on how the new information will impact doctor–patient relationships.

Conversely, dominance ("D") and conscientiousness ("C") types may be more task-focused, so the instructor could also relate the new information to how it will impact their problem solving, such as how to speed diagnosis or recovery.

## Section summary: personality types

The personality types of audience members will be diverse and can be classified by such systems as the DiSC profile, which includes four types: dominance, influence, steadiness, and conscientiousness. By knowing what different personality styles seek from a learning experience, an instructor can effectively reach the greatest number of attendees with his or her message.

# Section 6

## Audience experience

Teaching adults (andragogy) differs from teaching children (pedagogy) in one very important way: when teaching adults, it is necessary to accommodate the experience adult learners possess (see BioBox 2-2.) Whereas children are relatively "blank slates," adults have years' worth of accumulated experiences, and their very identities are based on these experiences. An adult's self-definition might involve his or her occupation, résumé, travels, training, and achievements (Knowles, 1970).

Because adults define themselves in terms of their experience, ideally, instructors will access that experience during their presentations. In fact, failing to acknowledge the learners' experience can leave learners feeling rejected. Conversely, drawing on their experience makes new information more meaningful for the learner. For an instructor, the audience's experience is an active resource that can help bring static material to life. Table 2-9 provides some tips for how an instructor can draw on audience experience.

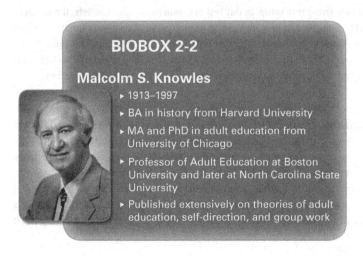

**BIOBOX 2-2**

**Malcolm S. Knowles**

- 1913–1997
- BA in history from Harvard University
- MA and PhD in adult education from University of Chicago
- Professor of Adult Education at Boston University and later at North Carolina State University
- Published extensively on theories of adult education, self-direction, and group work

**TABLE 2-9:** Sample strategies for drawing on audience experience

| Questions | Specific: "Has anyone here had a patient who..." Room poll: "Raise your hands if your patients have reported..." |
|---|---|
| Referential statements | "Patients may worry that _____, but this slide shows that..." <br><br>"Prescribers may think that _____, but this information suggests that..." <br><br>"You all know how insurance companies handle this, so a workaround is ..." |

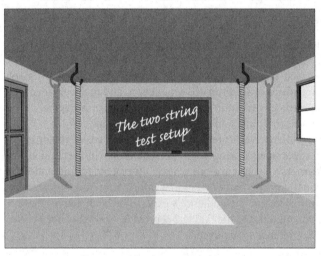

Figure 2-11. **The two-string test setup.** In this test of creativity and fixed beliefs, the subject's task is to connect two long strings that are hanging from a ceiling. The subject cannot reach both strings at the same time. A chalkboard is supplied to allow the subject to sketch out possibilities. The solution is to tie the eraser to one string and set it in motion, then stretch the second string toward the swinging string, catch the swinging string, and tie the two strings together.

The downside of dealing with experienced audiences is that adults have fixed habits and beliefs and are less open-minded than younger learners (Knowles, 1970). Lifetime experiences include misconceptions, biases, prejudices, and preferences that an instructor may have to overcome to impart knowledge. Evidence that experience can be a hindrance is supplied by the classic two-string test (Maier, 1931), shown in Figure 2-11. This test requires subjects to think about a familiar object in a new way – in this case, the eraser and string become a pendulum. Because experienced subjects habitually think of an eraser as only an eraser, they have difficulty with this test. Such "functional fixity" increases with education, as shown in Figure 2-12.

**TABLE 2-10**: Sample strategies for overcoming functional fixity in audiences

| | |
|---|---|
| **Old information, new use** | An instructor can ask learners if they know about the approval history of a relevant drug. The instructor can start off with something such as asking someone to name a drug initially approved for depression. The instructor can then ask for the learners to name other approved indications that came later (anxiety, pain, fibromyalgia, etc.). |
| **Historical but illogical reasons** | If trying to introduce a new practice, an instructor can help learners examine why they use old practices. For instance, if dosing or diagnosis was always done in a certain way, do the learners know why? Can anyone name the first use of the practice? |
| **Ideal but impractical solutions** | Before introducing new information, an instructor can ask learners to brainstorm ideal (if not practical) solutions to the problem being addressed. Could a brain implant or a trained parasite fix the problem? Thinking up impractical but useful ideas could open learners' minds to new information. |

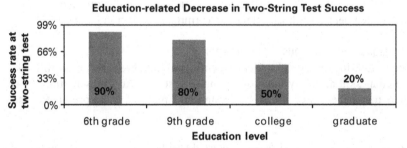

Figure 2-12. **Education-related decrease in success rate at the two-string test.** The rate of successful solving of the two-string test declined with education level. Study researchers suggested that this outcome was due to the fact that education inculcates rigid thinking in learners. (Dacey, 1989)

To overcome functional fixity, an instructor may have to encourage learners to think in new ways. Simply getting audience members to acknowledge that they harbor fixed beliefs, and getting them to examine why they hold those beliefs, may make them more accepting of new information. Some techniques for helping audiences break free of biases are given in Table 2-10.

### Section summary: audience experience

Adult medical audiences have a wealth of relevant experience. Drawing on audience experience can add impact to a presentation, whereas neglecting it can hinder the learners' receptivity to the instructor's message.

## Section 7

### Audience self-assessment

An effective medical educator will know not only where the audience members have been (their experience) but also where they are (their current knowledge level). Moreover, making learners aware of their current learning stage can aid in improving their knowledge and performance. Because adult learners perceive of themselves as being self-directed, they can become resentful in the traditional educational context, in which the teacher tells the audience what to learn. If society or the instructor has sufficient power to punish the audience for not learning – for example, by causing physicians to lose their licenses or preventing students from obtaining their degrees – then the learners will grudgingly submit to studying. However, learners are more deeply motivated to learn when they see the need to learn for their own purposes (Knowles, 1970). By guiding audience members to discover their own need for learning, an instructor can help them become enthusiastic about (instead of just resigned to) their role as learners.

One technique that aids an instructor in understanding the knowledge level of audience members is to classify stages of learning, as shown in Figure 2-13.

### Unconscious and conscious incompetents

"Unconscious incompetent" audience members are not even aware that they lack a particular skill and may unwittingly make mistakes. At a presentation, these learners may believe they already understand the material being presented; if so,

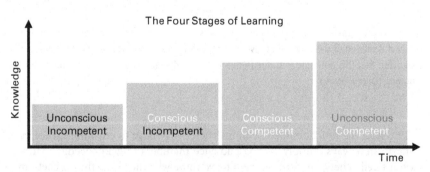

Figure 2-13. **The four stages of learning.** This figure shows one way to describe stages of learning as knowledge increases with time. (Howell, 1982)

they will pay little attention to the instructor. The leader can help them understand that they may be wrong in believing that they are already competent. For instance, medical learners may know that a certain medicine must be dosed with food, but they may not know what kind of food and why. The instructor can help the learners to realize they have more to learn by posing questions such as the following:

1. Does the drug upset an empty stomach, or does food aid the drug's absorption?
2. Is the dosage recommendation based on fat content in the food (for a lipid-soluble drug), or is it based only on gastrointestinal transit time?
3. How much food and what kind of food should be recommended?

Asking these questions can help learners realize that they do not really know what they think they know – they are "unconscious incompetents." By asking questions, the leader can help raise learner awareness to the level of "conscious incompetents." At this level, audience members know they lack knowledge and have the desire to correct the information gap.

## Conscious and unconscious competents

Conscious competents can perform a task, but only by thinking carefully about every aspect of it. For example, physicians may know that they should monitor plasma levels of a drug, but they may need to refer to guidelines to interpret lab results. By contrast, an unconscious competent could see the lab result and immediately know whether the level was appropriate. If information is imparted in a memorable way during a presentation – such as by means of a mnemonic or other memory tool – a conscious competent will be able to recall the explanation to perform the task at hand.

## Raising awareness

The instructor's role in the four stages of audience learning is given in Figure 2-14. As the figure illustrates, it will be advantageous to the instructor to raise the audience members' awareness of their current learning stage before attempting to impart knowledge. Information cannot be readily forced onto learners. So, rather than launching into a presentation, an instructor can first help audience members to be more receptive by helping them to understand their current level of knowledge about the presentation topics. Every audience can be made up of participants at each of the four stages of learning. Often, a participant can move only one stage forward at a single presentation. That is, those who are unconscious incompetents certainly go from ignorant bliss to a rude awakening – often immediately at the beginning of the presentation, as a result of just perusing the title and scanning the handout. Although that may be the extent of learning for those individuals for that session, this learning can be quite motivating for them to get to work gaining competence at a later date in the topics they now know that they do not know. To paraphrase the famous statement of former Secretary of Defense Donald Rumsfeld, these individuals have progressed from the "unknown unknowns" to the "known unknowns."

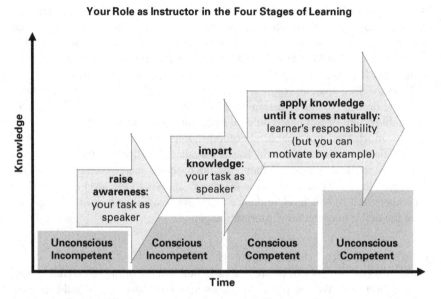

**Your Role as Instructor in the Four Stages of Learning**

Figure 2-14. **The role of the instructor in the four stages of learning.** This figure summarizes the instructor's role in the four stages of learning. The instructor will want to raise awareness (left arrow) before he or she can impart knowledge (center arrow).

Those who already know about their knowledge gaps – the conscious incompetents – with effort can go from ignorance to competence after attending a single well-designed presentation. Repetition and review at a later date, however, may be necessary to master and retain the information. Those who already have competence can go to a deeper understanding and a higher degree of retention of the material with another exposure to it (a review) in order to attain mastery at the level of "unconscious competence." It is an advantage for the instructor to know the level of competence of most in the audience before starting, but an instructor can also assume that, if there is something for all four quadrants of the typical audience, a wide breadth of participants will benefit from the presentation.

Although this section discusses the topics of competence and incompetence, an instructor certainly will not want to tell audience members that they are incompetent. Similarly, instructors generally will want to avoid threatening external sanctions, such as poor grades or even disapproval, because this approach will not aid learning. Adults are more motivated to learn when they self-diagnose a lack of some specific knowledge they need to achieve their own goals. Therefore, the instructor can help audience members to experience a feeling of dissatisfaction about their current knowledge and then help them to measure the gap between their present competency and the level of an ideal physician (Knowles, 1970). Some strategies instructors can use in encouraging self-assessment are given in Table 2-11.

| **TABLE 2-11:** Sample strategies instructors can use to encourage audience self-assessment | |
| --- | --- |
| **Refer to patient questions** | "If a patient asked you about this, would you know the exact answer, or would you be forced to resort to generalizations?"<br><br>"If a patient was worried about weight gain as a side effect, would you know which drugs are least likely to cause it?" |
| **Refer to colleagues' debates** | "If a colleague claims _____, would you be able to defend your position?" |
| **Refer to difficulties in diagnosing or prescribing** | "If presented with this possible differential diagnosis, would you know how to isolate the true condition?"<br><br>"If presented with a case like this, would you be forced to send the patient to a specialist?"<br><br>"If you wanted to prescribe this drug, would you know what dosage to give and which patients need dosage adjustments?" |
| **Identify ideal behaviors (which audience members may lack)** | "An experienced clinician can diagnose this condition within five minutes by asking the right questions."<br><br>"A knowledgeable psychiatrist always measures thyroid levels before prescribing an antidepressant." |

### Section summary: audience self-assessment
Adult learners are motivated to learn when they self-diagnose a need for knowledge. By helping audience members discover their own need for learning, instructors can cause them to be enthusiastic about (instead of just resigned to) their role as learners.

## Section 8

### Practical application

Medical learners are busy adults. They do not have much use for abstract knowledge or bits of arcana. Information is most valuable to them when they can see how knowing the material will benefit them in the immediate future. This is sometimes called the "what's in it for me" attitude. Learners benefit when new concepts are

**TABLE 2-12:** Sample strategies for emphasizing practical application

| Adult Desire | Application in a Presentation |
|---|---|
| **To gain something** | "This information will be crucial in helping you pass your certification exams." |
| | "If you learn this, you will be able to treat a wider range of patients instead of needing to refer them to specialists." |
| | "This information will help you gain continuing medical education credits." |
| **To be something** | "You can be mistake-free when treating this condition if you remember these points." |
| | "You will be respected by your colleagues if you know this information." |
| **To do something** | "You will be able to diagnose this condition in-house if you remember this information." |
| | "You will be able to prescribe the correct dosage of this medication if you remember this information." |
| **To save something** | "This information will save you time in diagnosis if you remember a few key points." |
| | "Following these guidelines will keep your actions legally defensible and will prevent increases in insurance costs." |

illustrated with specific, useful examples. Instructors can also help learners by providing opportunity for the learners to rehearse how they will use the knowledge in their everyday lives (Knowles, 1970).

During a discussion of practical applications of new information, it is useful to consider four motivations of adult learners (Lorge, 1947):

- adults want to gain something
- adults want to be something
- adults want to do something
- adults want to save something.

Some examples of how to address these four desires are given in Table 2-12.

### Section summary: practical application

Adult medical learners are less interested in abstract knowledge and more interested in useful information. By helping audiences imagine using facts from a presentation, the instructor can motivate them to listen, learn, and remember.

## Section 9

### Cultural diversity

Modern medicine is a global affair. Medical instructors are often invited to give talks at international locations, and most local audiences contain members of various cultures. Even if medical audience members all share the instructor's culture and ethnicity, they may treat patients from different backgrounds. A presentation that is successful at home may be ineffective abroad or may have reduced impact with different audiences.

It is often useful for an instructor to cast a critical eye on his or her data and consider them from the point of view of international audiences. Some issues to consider are presented in Table 2-13.

In addition to considering the ethnic implications of the medical data, the instructor will want to monitor his or her speech habits when speaking to multi-cultural audiences. It may be necessary to speak more slowly or articulate more clearly. Certain gestures or jokes may be ill-received. The culture of the audience

| TABLE 2-13: Medical presentation issues with cultural diversity | |
| --- | --- |
| **Presentation Elements** | **Ethnicity Considerations to Add** |
| **Study populations** | Are you presenting data from an all-white (or mostly white) patient population? What percentage of the population matches the ethnicity of your audience? Is there a replication of the study centered on the ethnicity of your audience? |
| **Diagnostic considerations** | When health care providers treat patients from certain cultures, will societal customs alter the symptom presentation? For example, a major depressive episode may involve complaints of nerves and headaches in Latino and Mediterranean cultures; of weakness, tiredness, or imbalance in Chinese and Asian cultures; of problems with the heart in Middle Eastern cultures; of being heartbroken among the Hopi. (DSM-IV-TR, 2005) |
| **Treatment recommendations** | Different medications may not be easily available in other countries; can learners suggest a replacement if needed? Do certain cultures have a reluctance toward certain treatment types? Do certain ethnicities metabolize the drug differently and therefore need specialized dosage recommendations? |

members can be researched before the presentation and an instructor may find it useful to ask his or her hosts questions about the culture of the audience.

### Section summary: cultural diversity

Medical audiences may include learners from a variety of cultures, and these learners may provide health care to patients of varying ethnicities. When an instructor addresses the issues of translating data and modifying behavior to suit various cultures, this can draw more learners into a presentation and make it more meaningful.

## Section 10

### Audience questions

Whether an instructor invites questions during the presentation or asks the audience to hold questions until the end, it is important to structure answers in a way that enhances learning. Even if the instructor does not know the answers to the audience's questions, he or she can make sure learners are satisfied by using the following strategies. One can even consider taking the approach of baseball great and folk philosopher Yogi Berra when he said, "I wish I had an answer to that because I am tired of answering that question."

### Acknowledge and repeat

First, the instructor can thank the learner for asking the question or for bringing up an interesting point, then repeat the question to the whole room. This step demonstrates to learners that the instructor welcomes interaction and it also ensures that everyone heard the question and is engaged in hearing the answer. In addition, it gives the instructor a chance to make sure he or she understood the question and time to gather his or her thoughts.

### Cite an authority

If a slide supports the answer to the question, the instructor can dial back to it on-screen (or mention that the slide is coming). If the instructor is answering from personal experience, he or she can also give a relevant resource (literature, Web site, etc.) in case the questioner wants to follow up on his or her own.

### Provide an answer or a resource

If the instructor is able to answer, he or she can do so. If unable to answer, he or she can tell the audience members where they can find the answer – either a literature resource, an electronic resource, or a human resource (such as a sales representative, if giving a promotional presentation).

### Suggest fair balance or provide disclaimers

Did the question or the answer negate some important consideration or obscure some important fact? If so, the instructor can respond by pointing out some of the following considerations: perhaps the questioner's comparisons were not head-to-head; perhaps the questioner cited studies that involve nonhuman subjects or small sample sizes; or perhaps the questioner needs to consider the issue of balancing risk with benefit.

One way to obtain closure is to check on whether a learner's question has been answered satisfactorily. If not, the instructor can follow up or offer to follow up after the presentation.

### Section summary: audience questions

Medical audiences include eager and sometimes combative questioners, but if an instructor can deal with questions appropriately, he or she will appear knowledgeable and helpful, which can enhance learning for the entire audience.

## Chapter summary

All audiences have the following:
- Tensions in the learning environment, including learner–instructor tension, learner-to-learner tension, and learner–material tension; addressing these tensions facilitates subsequent learning
- A finite attention span, which can be accommodated with the format of a presentation
- Members who may tend toward different types of learning, including
  - visual, auditory, reading/writing, or kinesthetic/tactile learning
  - divergent or convergent thinking
- A diversity of personality types – including those with characteristics of dominance, influence, steadiness, and conscientiousness – that may require the instructor to tailor presentation delivery accordingly

Medical learners are a unique audience, with:
- Experience that can be incorporated into a presentation
- A possible unawareness or misapprehension of their current level of learning (which the instructor can change)
- A need to know how information from a presentation can be applied in practical ways in the future
- Different cultural backgrounds and exposure to patients with various ethnicities
- A multitude of potentially difficult questions, which an instructor can be prepared to handle effectively even without knowing the answer

## Progress check

Write down your answers in the pages provided in the back of the book or on a separate piece of paper so that you can retake this test periodically without bias from your previous markings. Check your answers against the key in the back of the book and record your score in the ledger at the end of this quiz.

1. Audiences experience the four tensions that follow; which topic should be addressed last? Tension involving:
   a. Material
   b. Environment
   c. Other learners
   d. The instructor
2. At the beginning of a presentation, how long is learners' attention span?
   a. 45–50 minutes
   b. 30–35 minutes
   c. 15–20 minutes
   d. 3–4 minutes
3. At the end of an hour-long presentation, how long is learners' attention span?
   a. 45–50 minutes
   b. 30–35 minutes
   c. 15–20 minutes
   d. 3–4 minutes
4. Most members of medical audiences are multimodal learners, with a majority preference for learning that includes which element?
   a. Auditory
   b. Visual
   c. Kinesthetic/tactile
   d. Reading/writing
5. Which types of learners may be hardest to reach in a traditional lecture or presentation format?
   a. Auditory
   b. Visual
   c. Kinesthetic/tactile
   d. Reading/writing
6. Which of the following is not true about thinking styles in medical audiences?
   a. More experienced audiences are more likely to be convergent thinkers
   b. More experienced audiences are more likely to be divergent thinkers
   c. Encouraging audiences to use both styles may yield more thorough instruction
   d. Medical audiences are mostly convergent thinkers
7. What key words do the four personality styles stand for?
   a. Developer, Influence, Supervisor, Conscientiousness
   b. Dominance, Influence, Steadiness, Conscientiousness
   c. Dominant, Inventive, Steadiness, Creative
   d. Dynamic, Industrious, Sociable, Conscientiousness
8. The "D"s in your audience want the instructor to
   a. Be friendly
   b. Use humor
   c. Get to the point
   d. Be precise and detailed

9. Compared to the general population, medical audiences have
   a. Perhaps more "D"s
   b. Perhaps more "S"s
   c. Unusually low levels of "C"s
10. The "i"s in an audience want the instructor to
   a. Publicly recognize their contributions
   b. Be logical and orderly
   c. Let them initiate
   d. Be precise and focused
11. An audience may have many years of experience relevant to a presentation. How should this affect the instructor's delivery?
   a. During the introduction, the instructor should ask listeners to suspend preconceptions and listen with an open mind
   b. When presenting new material, the instructor should mention or ask about their experience with similar material
   c. The instructor can expect that audience members' breadth of knowledge will allow them greater capacity for openness to new ideas
12. The audience member who might be most eager to hear new information is
   a. The unconscious incompetent
   b. The conscious incompetent
   c. The conscious competent
   d. The unconscious competent
13. Medical audiences are perhaps most interested in which kind of information?
   a. Detailed and esoteric knowledge, above the comprehension level of laymen
   b. Abstract principles and broad generalization of concepts
   c. Specific application of information to practical examples
14. Which of the following is true about fielding questions from an audience?
   a. The instructor should answer as quickly as possible
   b. It is okay for the instructor to admit if he or she does not know the answer
   c. The instructor should give finality to the answer to seal off further debate
   d. Repeating the question will make the audience think the instructor is stalling

## Performance ledger

| Assessment | Date | Scoring |
| --- | --- | --- |
| 1 | | # correct answers: percent correct answers (divide by 14): |
| 2 | | # correct answers: percent correct answers (divide by 14): |
| 3 | | # correct answers: percent correct answers (divide by 14): |
| 4 | | # correct answers: percent correct answers (divide by 14): |
| 5 | | # correct answers: percent correct answers (divide by 14): |

## Performance self-assessment

Photocopy this page or write down your answers on a separate piece of paper so that you can retake this assessment periodically without bias from your previous markings. Record your score in the ledger on the next page.

| | 1 Poor, or Strongly Disagree | 2 Fair, or Disagree | 3 Average, or Neutral | 4 Good, or Agree | 5 Great, or Strongly Agree |
|---|---|---|---|---|---|
| **Structuring the learning environment** | | | | | |
| 1. I routinely assess and address tensions in the learning environment before I begin my presentations. | ☐ | ☐ | ☐ | ☐ | ☐ |
| 2. I routinely incorporate change-ups into my presentations. | ☐ | ☐ | ☐ | ☐ | ☐ |
| **Knowing your audience** | | | | | |
| 3. I am aware of the different learning styles (visual, auditory, reading/writing, kinesthetic/tactile) in my audience, and I try to cater to them. | ☐ | ☐ | ☐ | ☐ | ☐ |
| 4. I am aware of the different thinking styles (divergent versus convergent) in my audience, and I try to encourage both kinds of thinking. | ☐ | ☐ | ☐ | ☐ | ☐ |
| 5. I am aware of the different personality styles (DiSC) in my audience, and I try to accommodate them. | ☐ | ☐ | ☐ | ☐ | ☐ |
| 6. I routinely draw on audience experience when making presentations. | ☐ | ☐ | ☐ | ☐ | ☐ |
| 7. I routinely encourage self-assessment to raise audience awareness of knowledge levels before presenting new information. | ☐ | ☐ | ☐ | ☐ | ☐ |
| 8. I routinely give practical applications for concepts I present. | ☐ | ☐ | ☐ | ☐ | ☐ |
| 9. I routinely incorporate cultural and ethnic considerations into my behavior and my data. | ☐ | ☐ | ☐ | ☐ | ☐ |

| Fielding questions | | | | | |
|---|---|---|---|---|---|
| 10. I seek clarification before answering questions. | ☐ | ☐ | ☐ | ☐ | ☐ |
| 11. I ensure resolution after answering questions. | ☐ | ☐ | ☐ | ☐ | ☐ |
| Total number of checkmarks per column: | – | – | – | – | – |

## Performance self-assessment score sheet

| Assessment | Date | Scoring | 1 | 2 | 3 | 4 | 5 |
|---|---|---|---|---|---|---|---|
| Sample | 23 July 2009 | # items with each score: | 1×1 | 3×2 | 3×3 | 3×4 | 2×5 |
| | | Value | 1 | 6 | 9 | 12 | 10 |
| | | Total score (sum of value line): 38 | | | | | |
| | | Percent success (divide score by maximum, 60): 63% | | | | | |
| 1 | | # items with each score: | ×1 | ×2 | ×3 | ×4 | ×5 |
| | | Value | | | | | |
| | | Total score (sum of value line): | | | | | |
| | | Percent success (divide score by maximum, 55): | | | | | |
| 2 | | # items with each score: | ×1 | ×2 | ×3 | ×4 | ×5 |
| | | Value | | | | | |
| | | Total score (sum of value line): | | | | | |
| | | Percent success (divide score by maximum, 55): | | | | | |
| 3 | | # items with each score: | ×1 | ×2 | ×3 | ×4 | ×5 |
| | | Value | | | | | |
| | | Total score (sum of value line): | | | | | |
| | | Percent success (divide score by maximum, 55): | | | | | |
| 4 | | # items with each score: | ×1 | ×2 | ×3 | ×4 | ×5 |
| | | Value | | | | | |
| | | Total score (sum of value line): | | | | | |
| | | Percent success (divide score by maximum, 55): | | | | | |

| Assessment | Date | Scoring | | | | | |
|---|---|---|---|---|---|---|---|
| 5 | | # items with each score: | ×1 | ×2 | ×3 | ×4 | ×5 |
| | | Value | | | | | |
| | | Total score (sum of value line): | | | | | |
| | | Percent success (divide score by maximum, 55): | | | | | |

# Executing the principles of adult learning in medical presentations

## Chapter overview

Chapter 3 examines how instructors can maximize effectiveness by balancing their presentation efforts between "what is said" and "how it is said." Constructing a successful educational presentation is similar to constructing any other object. The job requires a combination of factors: namely, having a plan plus having the required tools and then applying the skilled use of those tools leads to a successful "build." This chapter explores an array of tools and how to use them to increase the success of presentations.

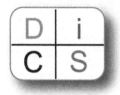

Personality affects both sides of the communication equation. A presenter's personality style will affect how he or she chooses to communicate with the audience. The various personalities represented in the audience will influence how the instructor's message is received. Because personality affects the way learners perceive an instructor, the instructor's ability to convey knowledge hinges in part upon personality. The key to effectiveness for an instructor is to know his or her own style and what strategies need to be employed to expand success across all **personality styles**. This chapter will discuss how knowing personality styles of oneself and one's audience (e.g. by using DiSC definitions) can allow an instructor to leverage his/her personality style to enhance the transmission of information.

Practice and preparation are critical keys to success. Understanding the components of preparation allows for the development of a thorough plan that can

be practiced. Practicing the "what" and "how" until it all becomes second nature facilitates exceptional presentations. This level of preparation is almost instantaneously recognized by an audience and increases an instructor's persuasiveness. It also allows the instructor the freedom to monitor the audience. The second section discusses how to use **preparation** to identify places to add emphasis and insert builds that will set up and then deliver an educational punch line, enabling better understanding and higher retention levels.

The use of words and sentence structure are important, but verbal and nonverbal behaviors can carry surprisingly more weight than the actual

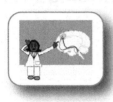

words. The section on **verbal and nonverbal behaviors** discusses how to use both verbal and nonverbal communication techniques to the greatest benefit. An effective instructor is able to identify places to add impact by using verbal and nonverbal behaviors and also knows how to avoid nonverbal messages that are conflicting or distracting.

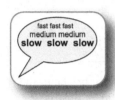

**Rate of speech** is a major factor that can be mastered to improve speaking effectiveness. In general, instructors need to work on slowing down. Speaking slowly may feel unnatural at first but can work to ensure that learners will comprehend information and take notes. Slower speech can even lend a perception that a topic is of great importance.

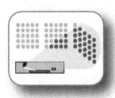

The last section discusses the **use of proxemics**. An instructor who knows the power of position and posture has the potential to be much more effective. This section explores this subset of communication science and provides the reader with insights that can significantly enhance any instructional endeavor they lead.

## Introduction

### Rationale and benefits

Every instructor wants to be remembered – as dynamic, as powerful, as professional, as intelligent, as whatever – but remembered. Medical educators also want the material to be remembered. The two goals go hand-in-hand.

To achieve these goals, instructors can usefully examine their own personalities in relationship to the personalities in the medical audience and determine which traits can contribute to improving communication across the various types represented. This chapter discusses strategies for optimum use of personality characteristics so that instructors can present themselves and the content they want to convey in the best possible way.

Every personality carries with it both advantages and challenges. Learning the various types and their corresponding traits enables instructors to utilize successful communication strategies with all types in their audiences. This chapter also provides some tips on how to practice more effectively. Dull repetition leads to a dull presentation; however, identifying places to add impact will pay off in better learning – whether through using builds in slides or through appropriate body language so that it comes most naturally. Even practicing the rate of speech is important and often neglected. Rate of speech is critical for audiences listening in English as a second language and for audience members listening to a simultaneous translation into their native language and not to the speaker.

## Section 1

## Personality

*If you can't imitate him, don't copy him.* (Yogi Berra)

The more an instructor is aware of his or her own personality, the better that instructor can relate to the different personalities found in any audience. The Myers-Briggs type assessment (Myers *et al.*, 1998) and the DiSC profile (Inscape, 1996) are excellent measures of personality. For information on how to obtain your DiSC profile, please call 1760–795-2005 ext 133. Many online resources are also readily available that give an in-depth personality analysis.

This section focuses on the personality types of instructors and examines useful strategies that can be used with each. These strategies are based on the instructor being aware of his or her own style and then knowing how to adapt that style to be more effective with each of the various styles in the audience. Also examined in this section are cues an instructor can look for to identify different types in an audience.

Instructors who have taken the DiSC personality profile can modulate presentation style based on the results of that profile.

### Modulating a "D" (dominance) personality
"D" type educators are at ease in a leadership role. They are rapid processors of information and decisive thinkers with good problem-solving skills. These qualities are favorable characteristics to possess. The quick pace and directness of a "D," while potentially beneficial, can cause the perception of coldness, impatience, and even intimidation. "D" types, in their drive for results, can become impersonal and demanding, especially when the perceived rate of progress is slower than they desire. To improve, a "D" will want to develop a greater level of patience, tone down directness, and ask a few more questions to create a more personable environment where people in the audience have the opportunity to offer some input into the presentation.

### Modulating an "i" (influence) personality
Instructors who are an "i" type are often good at inspiring others. They are also very enthusiastic and known for their ability to connect with others.

These are all great qualities for an instructor. However, "i"s can be pulled off topic by sharing personal experiences that may not be relevant to the content being covered. An "i" type may not include enough detail to be clear when giving directions. Follow-through and organization are not strengths of this type. To take steps to improve, "i"s will want to be more organized in their general approach to things and be more specific when giving directions. Developing processes and systems can significantly raise the level of accomplishment for "i" types.

## Modulating an "S" (steadiness) personality

For an "S" type instructor, strengths might include empathy and sensitivity to audience needs. "S" types are methodical when approaching a task and are consistent in their leadership style and their overall performance. On the limitation side, they can be somewhat indecisive and resistant to change, even when that change is perceived as good. This characteristic means that "S"s may be slower to implement changes when needed. They may shy away from conflict, as they are strongly oriented to positive relationships. Taking steps to improve for an "S" include becoming more assertive and direct when needed. Working harder to understand and then implement change can also bring about higher levels of effectiveness for "S" types.

## Modulating a "C" (conscientiousness) personality

One of the great things that can be said about "C" type instructors is that they have very high standards that they hold themselves to as well as others. They are driven by accuracy and thus their presentation materials are extremely accurate and well researched. "C"s usually have a reputation for fairness and being able to keep a confidence among their peers. Their high standards, fairness, and trustworthiness are beneficial characteristics. The limitations for "C"s are that some audiences would perceive them as perfectionist and perhaps even aloof in their interactions with people. To improve presentations, "C"s can work on accepting personality types different from themselves, include more discussion with the audience members, and be a little less focused on detail.

## Observable cues for type identification

An instructor can use the cues described here to help identify the different personalities in an audience. As discussed in the next section on preparation, arriving early has many benefits, one of which is that it enables the educator to have the time to make some of the identifications described below.

### Cues for identifying "D"s

"D"s are one of the easiest types to identify. They walk into a room as if on a mission, choose their seat quickly, and have a "no nonsense" demeanor. They are direct when addressing someone and speak with a faster rate of speech. When they interact with someone, it usually wouldn't be described as personable.

*Cues for identifying "i"s*
The "i" types are easy to recognize as well. They too are a little quicker-paced and in fact might be described as energetic. They, however, are more concerned with seeking out someone to interact with before choosing where they would sit. They are very personable and connect easily with others.

*Cues for identifying "S"s*
"S"s may not be as easy to identify as quickly as the "D"s and "i"s but they have definite behaviors that help in their identification. The "S" types enter the room at a much slower pace, almost tentatively, and perhaps stand just inside the doorway and look around the room for a moment or two. Their movements would not be as deliberate and they may take a while deciding where they are going to sit. They wouldn't seek out interaction but would be open to it.

*Cues for identifying "C"s*
"C"s, like the "S"s, move at a more moderate pace. They might come into the room checking paperwork having to do with the meeting, looking at their materials, and even moving to various sections of the room as they evaluate the best area to sit in. They may check a list or prepare their "area" with careful placement of each item.

## Section summary: personality
Personality affects both sides of the communication equation. It influences the way the instructor will choose to communicate and the way the message will be received. An instructor's knowledge and accommodation of this factor is proportional to the success he or she will have transmitting the information in the presentation. If medical educators know their own personality style and what strategies to use with other styles, and if they can identify the composition of their audience, then they can be highly effective in helping others learn and retain the information presented.

# Section 2

## Preparation

*If you don't know where you're going, you'll wind up somewhere else.* (Yogi Berra)

As was stated earlier in the book, "it's all in the setup." The setup in this case is what and how to prepare. The desired outcome or learning objective is the first stone to lay in the foundation of any presentation. The next step incorporates a "participant focus" to establish the best way to accomplish the objective through the eyes of the learner. When the instructor is the builder of the presentation, he or she can plan and assemble the presentation that best facilitates the learning.

To be truly effective in front of an audience, an instructor will not only know the material being presented but also will know the sequence of the information or how the story is told. Then the serious medical educator will be able to identify places to incorporate preview and review or a question, an anecdote, or various other techniques that either advance learning or maintain audience engagement. By thoroughly knowing the material, how it is assembled, techniques, and timing, instructors are able to focus on tailoring the presentation to the audience.

## Multimedia preparation and builds

Instructors who understand and enjoy using multimedia tools, especially PowerPoint builds, can determine during the organization of a medical presentation where in the presentation these may be most relevant. Builds allow for parceling out information that would be overwhelming all at once, but instructors will want to be well acquainted with the builds so they can set up a punch line and then reveal it, as discussed in Chapter 1. Some suggestions for helpful builds are given in Table 1-1 in Chapter 1 and in Table 3-1. However, excessive builds will tie the instructor to the remote control or to the computer. Instructors will also want to avoid flashy or distracting effects. The goal is to enhance learning, not detract from it.

## Practiced style elements and audience perceptions

An instructor's preparation includes more than just reviewing the factual specifics of a presentation, as was previously discussed. Audience members will judge a presentation on more than just the data; as shown in Figure 3-1, audiences also consider an instructor's persuasiveness and other contributing elements (column labels). An instructor's practiced style elements (row labels) influence the perceptions of audience members.

- Fluency is important and, as shown in the diagram, influences the perceptions of competence, composure, and sociability as well as persuasiveness. Fluency is improved by practicing.
- Lack of preparation forces an instructor to read from slides, increasing the likelihood of reduced tonal inflection or variance. This performance short-coming negatively impacts perceived character, competence, sociability, and persuasiveness.
- Just as in conversation with an individual, the instructor's eye contact with audience members is one of the most influential aspects of delivery. Proper preparation and familiarity with the material allow the presenter to maximize the level of direct eye contact and minimize visual disconnects with the audience. As evidenced in the chart, poor eye contact would call the instructor's character into question, which makes the message suspect as well. In Section 3 of this chapter, the portion on nonverbal behaviors contains some important suggestions to enhance an instructor's ability to raise the level of eye contact.
- Smiling helps, even if only during the time the instructor is welcoming the audience; if a presentation topic is no smiling matter, during the rest of the presentation the instructor can use other more appropriate facial expressions.

| **TABLE 3-1:** Helpful builds for medical presentations | |
|---|---|
| **Graphs** | Instructors can bring in the non-data ink first, such as the axis, without the bars or lines representing the data ink. This allows time for a description of what is being measured and how. Once the audience members understand the point of the study, the instructor can click to reveal the results. |
| **Anatomy** | Instructors can show an unlabeled cell/tissue/organ/system first, then introduce each label on a click, starting with the most easily recognized feature and moving to successively subtler features. Similarly, it is effective to show features of a healthy system first, then click to reveal disordered, dysregulated, or diseased features. |
| **Mode of Action** | Instructors can show the drug target first (receptor, antigen, nucleic acid, etc.) in its usual biological context and explain the predrug functioning system. Then instructors can click to introduce the drug and show its downstream effects with an appropriate number of successive clicks. |
| **Tables** | Instructors can bring in the headers first and describe what was being measured and how (non-data ink). Then instructors can introduce data row by row or column by column (whichever way presents the most important comparisons—i.e., the data ink). |

Notice that a smile touches every category on the persuasiveness side of the chart.

- Illustrator gestures, such as pointing at an important piece of information, are indirectly related to persuasiveness and can help an audience follow the information being presented.
- Preparation will help lessen nervousness, reduce fidgeting, and prevent body tension, resulting in greater persuasiveness.
- Using body movement – instead of clinging to the podium – shows that an instructor is comfortable with the presentation. When an instructor occasionally moves to a new vantage point, this ensures that different audience members can see the instructor.

Many of the items scored as important for persuasiveness are nonverbal behaviors – body language. Such nonverbal behaviors are discussed in the pages that follow.

| Your style elements | Qualities the audience perceives | | | | |
|---|---|---|---|---|---|
| | **Persuasion** | Sociability | Competence | Character | Composure |
| Fluency | ● | ● | ● | ● | ● |
| Pitch variety | ● | ● | ● | ● | |
| Eye contact | ● | ● | | ● | |
| Smiling | ● | ● | ● | ● | ● |
| Facial expressiveness | ● | ● | ● | | |
| Illustrator gestures | | ● | | | |
| Object fidgeting (less) | ● | | | | |
| Body tension (less) | | ● | | | |
| Body movement | | ● | | | |

Figure 3-1. **Evidence of preparation increases persuasiveness.** To generate these data, researchers videotaped 30 undergraduates delivering a required persuasive speech. An audience of their peers (*N* = 30) rated the instructors' credibility and persuasiveness. Two trained coders scored the instructors' nonverbal behaviors on a 7-point differential scale. Twenty-two nonverbal behaviors were scored; the nine shown in this figure are those found to have statistically significant importance. (Burgoon *et al.*, 1990)

### Section summary: preparation
Evidence of preparation increases persuasiveness and allows an instructor the freedom to monitor the audience. Instructors can use preparation to identify places to add emphasis and insert builds. Once those accommodations are completed, practice can insure effective performance.

## Section 3

### Verbal and nonverbal behaviors

*What you do speaks so loud that I cannot hear what you say.* (Ralph Waldo Emerson)

### What is said versus how it is said
Despite the importance of medical data, this book has been emphasizing that there is much more to giving a presentation than just the words describing the data. Pioneering experiments by Dr. Albert Mehrabian attempted to quantify the importance of elements of a presentation such as presentation style, voice fluency, and body language.
● In the first experiment (Mehrabian and Ferris, 1967), facial expressions communicating like, dislike, or neutrality were photographed. A neutral word ("maybe") was selected by 25 subjects, and voices communicating like, neutrality, or dislike were recorded speaking the word. A second group of 17 subjects assessed these independent facial and vocal communications. Then, a third group of 20 subjects was presented with facial–vocal

**Quantified Impact of Verbal and Nonverbal Behaviors**

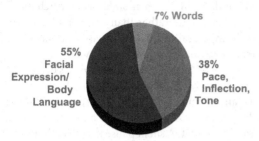

7% Words

55%
Facial
Expression/
Body
Language

38%
Pace,
Inflection,
Tone

Figure 3-2. **Quantified impact of verbal and nonverbal behaviours.** (Mehrabian, 1971)

combinations and were given these directions: "Imagine that the person that you see and hear (A) is looking at and talking to another person (B). For each presentation, indicate on the scale what you think A's attitude is towards B."

- In the second experiment (Mehrabian and Wiener, 1967), 45 subjects selected words with positive, neutral, or negative connotations. Positive words were "honey," "thanks," and "dear"; neutral words were "maybe," "really," and "oh"; and negative words were "don't," "brute," and "terrible." Contribution of tone and content were assessed by 10 subjects each. Finally, 10 subjects decoded the message when tone and word were presented together, similar to the first experiment.

The results of these studies were pooled to yield the results shown in Figure 3-2.

The results of these experiments suggest that audience perceptions of a message are based very little on the simple content of the spoken words. To summarize this research in an aphorism, it is not what is said (only 7%), it is how it's said (93%). These numerical values may be approximate, but the relative importance should hold in most situations. Therefore, instructors can definitely use body language and vocal tone to their advantage, while avoiding verbal and nonverbal behaviors that work against them.

## Verbal behaviors

Here are some principles of vocal tone and verbal behavior.

- Avoid conflicting combinations of tone and content. For example, with sarcasm, words oppose tone, and impact is reduced. Similarly, if instructors say they are open to questions but fold their arms over their chest, this body language conveys that the instructor is actually closed off from audience interaction.
- Use additive combinations whenever possible. If an instructor tells the audience that a piece of information is exciting, the vocal tone used can convey "excitement!" If a certain bar on a graph is important, the instructor can point at it or use his or her hands to measure the difference between that bar and the other bars.
- Because vocal quality is so important, instructors can try to keep their heads up to avoid compressing the vocal cords. It is helpful if instructors therefore do not

rely on notes that will force their heads down for reading. As mentioned earlier, it is more likely that instructors today will use their slides as a crutch and as speaker notes, possibly talking to the screen rather than to the audience, and depending upon amplification, losing vocal quality. Instructors can also stand up straight to allow for the greatest resonance in the chest cavity.

- Avoid fill speech. Fill speech – using words such as "um" or "ah" – is evidence of lack of fluency. Most speakers are entirely unaware of their own fill speech. Few things are more off-putting to an audience. However, few speaker flaws are potentially more remediable by a speaker who is attentive and who monitors this problem and knows how to overcome it. A silent pause to collect thoughts is not only less distracting to an audience but can actually add emphasis to the idea spoken.
- Identify words that should be emphasized. For example, an instructor who wants the audience to focus on the role of dopamine in depression might say, "Clinicians often prescribe selective serotonin reuptake inhibitors for depression, but it's DOPAMINE we need to target in a case like this."

### Nonverbal behaviors

In considering nonverbal behaviors, it may be helpful to consider categories established by pioneering researchers in semiotics (Ekman and Friesen, 1969). An instructor can always keep in mind that in the worldwide forum of modern medicine, body language elements in these categories can be interpreted differently by members of different cultures. Categories of nonverbal behavior include the following.

1. **Emblems** can be translated into words. Examples are the "okay" sign, the V-for-victory sign, and the thumbs-up sign.
2. **Illustrators** are gestures to add emphasis, such as pointing to an element on a slide.
3. **Affect displays** are nonverbal emotional displays. For example, nervousness may be conveyed via hand wringing or fidgeting.
4. **Regulators** are nonverbal acts that initiate, maintain, or terminate speech. For example, when an instructor nods as learners ask questions, this encourages the learners.
5. **Adaptors** are acts related to satisfaction of bodily needs. For example, an instructor may be shifting his or her weight only to be more comfortable, but this motion may be distracting to learners.

Illustrators are one of the most useful nonverbal behaviors during a presentation, and regulators are helpful for inviting interaction from the audience. Emblems can be useful in "acting out" parts of the presentation.

Instructors may want to minimize affect displays and adaptors. Also, because body language is so important, instructors will want to avoid hiding behind a podium where audiences can't see half their body.

Instructors can try practicing a presentation in front of a mirror and categorizing nonverbal behaviors – are they helpful or distracting? Do the nonverbal behaviors call attention to the learning or to the instructor? Examples of adding

| **TABLE 3-2**: Helpful nonverbal behaviors for medical presentations | |
|---|---|
| **Emblems** | Gestures translate data into actions: |
| | ▸ Using both hands to measure a large difference between two bars on a graph or pinching fingers together emphasizes a large or tiny difference between bars. |
| | ▸ If a graph slopes sharply up or levels off over time, this can be emphasized by sloping a hand to match the trend. |
| | ▸ Tapping out a fast heart rate when describing one condition and slowly tapping out the converse condition emphasizes the difference between the two conditions. |
| | ▸ If an anatomical location "lights up" on a scan under certain conditions, flashing a hand will highlight the active condition. |
| **Illustrators** | Pointing to an important statistic or anatomical location reinforces the verbal content. |
| **Regulators** | Open and welcoming gestures invite contributions from learners. |

helpful nonverbal behavior to a presentation are given in Table 3-2. Instructors can play back audio recordings of a presentation, evaluating voice modulation, fill speech, and modulation of pace for emphasis. Better yet, instructors can play back video, in which both verbal and nonverbal characteristics can be reviewed for future improvement.

One of the most important and powerful nonverbal behaviors is use of eye contact. Eye contact by the instructor is significantly associated with audience perceptions of the instructor's character, sociability, and persuasiveness (Burgoon *et al.*, 1990). Greater levels of eye contact by the instructor when he or she is giving instructions improve performance by the learner (Fry and Smith, 1975). The mechanism for gaze-facilitated learning may be partially due to eye contact acting as an arousal stimulus to the learner, increasing attention and therefore facilitating the learner's encoding of information (Fullwood and Doherty-Sneddon, 2006). The converse also may be true: gaze aversion can decrease learning. Individuals who avoid eye contact may be perceived as defensive, evasive, and/or inattentive (Fullwood and Doherty-Sneddon, 2006). Audiences may form a negative impression of these eye-averting instructors, and therefore learners may be less inclined to listen to what those instructors have to say (Fullwood and Doherty-Sneddon, 2006). A quantified effect of eye contact on learning is shown in Figure 3-3.

An instructor should work to maintain the highest level of eye contact with the audience members. An instructor speaking to a large audience on a large stage will find that using a confidence monitor is helpful. These monitors are typically

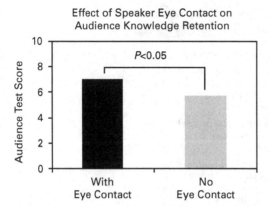

Figure 3-3. **Effect of instructor eye contact on audience knowledge retention.** Participants (*N* = 32, each tested individually) viewed recordings of an instructor giving a presentation, either without eye contact or with eye contact (30% to 32% of time looking into camera). Afterward, participants were tested on recall of the presentation (maximum score=21). Compared to the gaze-aversion condition, viewers retained information better when the presentation was given with direct eye contact. (Fullwood and Doherty-Sneddon, 2006)

42-inch flat screens placed strategically in front of the instructor so that visual references to the content being presented can be accomplished with minimal loss of eye contact. In a smaller audience setting, the instructor can use a laptop in much the same way, placing it far away enough so as not to stare down at it but close enough so it is easily read.

### Section summary: verbal and nonverbal behaviors

An instructor's nonverbal behaviors can carry even more weight than his or her words, so consider the impact of body language, eye contact, and vocal emphasis carefully. Polishing a presentation can mean identifying places where adding emphasis can be done with nonverbal behaviors, while avoiding nonverbal messages that are conflicting or distracting.

## Section 4

### The rate of speech

*I'm not talking too fast – you're listening too slow!* (B. Mitchel Reed, Disc Jockey)

Most lectures are presented at a rate of 100 to 180 words per minute (wpm); these are divided into slow (100 wpm), medium (150 wpm), and fast (180 wpm) for Figure 3-4 (Robinson *et al.*, 1997). The faster rates of speech can exceed an adult learner's listening rate, which is around 150 to 175 wpm (Figure 3-4). When learners are also taking notes, they can only comprehend about 135 wpm (Robinson *et al.*, 1997), and even more information can be missed (Figure 3-4). Therefore, an instructor may

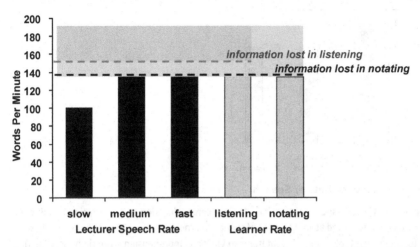

Figure 3-4. **Lecturer speech rate versus learner comprehension and note-taking rate.** All information above the gray dashed line is lost to the learner who is listening; thus, some information imparted by a fast-talking lecturer is lost to listeners. Information above the black dashed line is lost to the learner who is taking notes; thus, information is lost when imparted by lecturers who speak either at a fast or medium rate. Only information by the slow-speaking lecturers is not lost on any learner. (Robinson *et al.*, 1997)

need to slow down to allow learners to keep up in their writing. By watching the audience members, an instructor will know to pause in a presentation until note takers finish writing and look up again to signify they're ready to continue learning.

Research has consistently shown that listening comprehension suffers as speaking rate increases (Robinson *et al.*, 1997). Learners also rate topics as more important when instructors speak more slowly, as shown in Figure 3-5. Therefore, speaking slowly imparts a perception of value to the topic and leads to greater comprehension of the material.

Intentionally speaking slowly can also aid in preventing the phenomenon known as "trail-off." Because people can think faster than they can speak, an instructor's thoughts might finish before the instructor gets to the end of a sentence or idea, and the instructor's volume drops substantially. This is detrimental to learners, who miss the end of the sentence and spend time trying to comprehend what was said – or even asking their neighbors what was said. Learners then miss the next idea presented.

## Section summary: the rate of speech

For an instructor, speaking slowly may feel unnatural at first, but it ensures that learners comprehend and can take notes on the information presented. Slower speech can even lend a perception of greater importance to the topic.

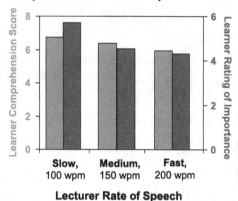

**Figure 3-5. Lecturer speech rate affects learner comprehension and perception of value.** A lecture was videotaped at various rates of speech. Learners (*N* =19 or 20 per group) watched the lecture and then took a quiz of eight items to yield a comprehension score (light gray bars). Learners also rated the topic in importance on a 10-point scale, with 10 being most important (dark gray bars). Slower speech rates by the instructor led to greater comprehension by the learners (main effect $P < 0.05$). Learners also rated the topic as more important when the instructor spoke more slowly (main effect $P < 0.01$). (Robinson *et al.*, 1997)

## Section 5

### The use of proxemics

This chapter has already pointed out that an instructor will want to step out from behind the podium. In small settings, an instructor can move to certain locations in the room to gain the attention of distant learners. Research by Edward T. Hall (BioBox 3-1) has shown that learners seated more than 10 feet away from the instructor can consider the instructor "public" (Figure 3-6), meaning they might not feel compelled to acknowledge the instructor's presence. They also might feel a certain intellectual distance from the message. If the instructor moves to a location within 9 feet of the learners, the "mandatory recognition distance" kicks in – that's when a person would have to acknowledge another on the street. If an instructor notices that learners in the back of the room are checking out mentally, the instructor can move within the 9-foot distance – into the "social-consultive" range – to get the learners' attention. However, an instructor will want to be careful to avoid infringing on someone's "personal space" (within 4 feet).

In a large venue, instructors can still put proxemics to work for them. The general proxemics principle of moving closer to those who are important can be utilized with even the largest of audiences. Shortening the distance between the instructor and a section of the audience has the same positive effect. Indeed, if an

## BIOBOX 3-1

### Edward T. Hall

- Born 1914
- BA in anthropology from University of Denver; PhD in anthropology from Columbia University
- Held positions at Washington School of Psychiatry, University of Denver, Bennington College, Harvard Business School, Illinois Institute of Technology, and Northwestern University
- Published many books on cross-cultural communication
- His innovative theories of proxemics (human perceptions of space) strongly influenced fields of anthropology and communication theory

**American Proxemic Perceptions**

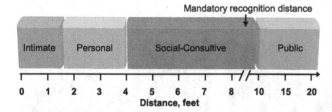

Figure 3-6. **American proxemic perceptions.** An instructor can move within 9 feet of learners so that a mandatory recognition distance kicks in, to get the learners' attention. An instructor will want to be careful, however, to avoid infringing on someone's personal space within 4 feet. (Hall, 1968)

instructor who is presenting to a large audience notices that learners in the back row are leaning back in the chairs or displaying other indicators of disengaging, the instructor can make eye contact with them and combine this with as little as a half step towards them. These actions can immediately cause the learners to sit up into a more active listening posture and become re-engaged in the presentation.

Another very effective action when an instructor is on a wide stage with a large audience is to choose three presentation positions – left, center, and right. By repositioning at intervals throughout the presentation, the instructor can equally distribute audience section attention. This is not to say that the instructor is in constant movement or paces across a stage, which many audience members will find distracting.

Instructors can make the effort throughout the presentation to stay aware of whether they are facing the audience, as shown in Figure 3-7. Instructors can also gauge the learners' line of sight to the screen and avoid blocking this. If an instructor moves periodically to new positions and angles, this will ensure that no groups of audience members are ignored and that everyone has a chance to see the slides.

Also, instructors can keep any visual disconnect to a minimum when turning away from the audience to gesture at a salient item of information, whether using a hand or a laser pointer.

A laser pointer may seem like a helpful tool, but overusing it might cause instructors to turn their backs on the audience too often (see Figure 3-8). Moreover, if an instructor uses the laser for long durations or to draw out long lines (such as underlining text), this can exaggerate any instability or shaking of the hands. Attention is drawn to the instructor's nervousness, not to the learning topics. Instructors will want to limit themselves to a brief, 2-second laser dot on the item of interest. If data slides appear to call for lengthy use of a laser, an instructor may want to look at reconstructing the slide with builds to help differentiate the data, following the suggestions in Chapter 1.

### Section summary: the use of proxemics
Because nonverbal behaviors are so important, instructors will want to make sure that they position themselves advantageously so that the learners' perception of the

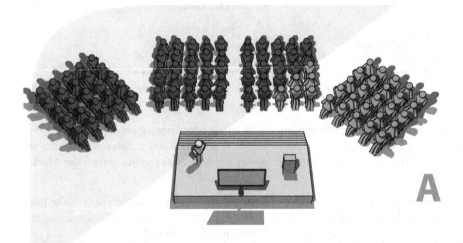

Figure 3-7. **Large-group proxemics.** In this figure, the white icon represents the instructor, and the gray field is the "receptive field" wherein audience members can see an instructor's face. In setting A, if instructors position themselves on the edge of the stage, they will want to be aware of those audience members (in light gray) who can't see their faces and body language. In setting B, if an instructor turns to read from a slide, fewer audience members (in dark gray) can see the instructor. Setting C shows one position that allows many audience members to see the instructor and could be duplicated left or right of the stage with the same results.

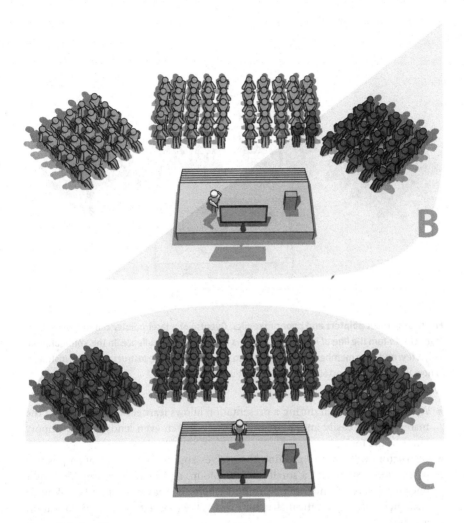

Figure 3-7. (cont.)

speaker is positively enhanced and so that eye contact with the audience members is optimized.

## Chapter summary

- Personality type affects presentation style; when instructors learn more about themselves, they are able to play up their strengths and modify behaviors that might be off-putting.
- Verbal and nonverbal behaviors carry even more weight than the actual words used; body language, eye contact, and vocal intonation can add emphasis and increase learning.

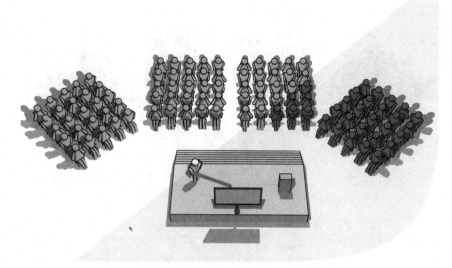

Figure 3-8. **Laser pointers and poor proxemics.** Overuse of a laser pointer can cause the instructor to turn the line of his or her shoulders away from the audience. In this configuration, only a few audience members (in dark gray) can see the front of the instructor and the instructor is now visually disconnected from a large portion of the audience.

- A slow rate of speech during a presentation allows learners to comprehend the material more easily and take notes; slower speech even lends greater importance to the topic.
- Instructors will want to position themselves appropriately to create a positive perception, whether in a small or large group, and to allow unimpeded sight lines to visuals. Maintaining a position where the maximum number of audience members can see the instructor's face is the most effective communication practice.

## Progress check

Write down your answers in the pages provided in the back of the book or on a separate piece of paper so that you can retake this test periodically without bias from your previous markings. Check your answers against the key in the back of the book and record your score in the ledger at the end of this quiz.

1. Instructors with a type "D" personality might need to
    a. Ask more questions of the audience
    b. Be more assertive and direct
    c. Be more open to change

2. Instructors with a type "i" personality might need to
   a. Be more specific when giving direction
   b. Try approaching things from a more organized standpoint
   c. Work to seem less aloof
   d. Both a and b
3. When presenting new data, instructors should
   a. Present the most compelling results first, then explain how they were obtained
   b. Present all relevant information at once so that audiences can get a comprehensive picture of your information
   c. Set up the backstory first, then reveal the results
4. Audiences are impacted most strongly by
   a. The content of the words
   b. Vocal tone, inflection, and pacing
   c. Facial expression and body language
5. Audience learning retention and audience perception of the instructor's persuasiveness can especially be increased by which instructor behavior?
   a. Eye contact
   b. Vocal pitch variety
   c. Illustrator gestures
   d. Smiling
6. Many types of body language are helpful to the audience, but which kind can be distracting?
   a. Emblems
   b. Illustrators
   c. Regulators
   d. Adaptors
7. Speaking at a pace that is comfortably brisk for the instructor
   a. Signifies to the audience that the instructor is confident of the topic
   b. Produces measurably higher attention levels in audience members, who can be lulled into boredom by slow speech
   c. Can preclude the ability of learners to comprehend the topic
   d. Both a and b
8. In small group, when the instructor moves within a certain distance he or she will break a "social" barrier. What is that target distance?
   a. < 4 feet
   b. < 9 feet
   c. < 11 feet
   d. < 13 feet
9. If an instructor is using a laser pointer, helpful behaviors include
   a. Underscoring lines of important text
   b. Drawing circles around important items
   c. Brief dots on relevant items
   d. All of the above

## Performance ledger

| Assessment | Date | Scoring |
|---|---|---|
| 1 | | # correct answers: |
| | | percent correct answers (divide by 9): |
| 2 | | # correct answers: |
| | | percent correct answers (divide by 9): |
| 3 | | # correct answers: |
| | | percent correct answers (divide by 9): |
| 4 | | # correct answers: |
| | | percent correct answers (divide by 9): |
| 5 | | # correct answers: |
| | | percent correct answers (divide by 9): |

## Performance self-assessment

Photocopy this page or write down your answers on a separate piece of paper so that you can retake this assessment periodically without bias from your previous markings. Record your score in the ledger on the next page.

| | 1 | 2 | 3 | 4 | 5 |
|---|---|---|---|---|---|
| | Poor, or Strongly Disagree | Fair, or Disagree | Average, or Neutral | Good, or Agree | Great, or Strongly Agree |
| **Before your presentations** | | | | | |
| 1. I am aware of my personality type and I try to modulate it to greatest effect for presentations. | | | | | |
| 2. I routinely practice my entire presentation before giving it. | | | | | |
| 3. My presentations contain appropriate builds to reveal information in high-impact ways. | | | | | |

| During your presentation | | | | | |
|---|---|---|---|---|---|
| 4. When feasible, I make eye contact with learners on all sides of the room equally. | | | | | |
| 5. I am aware of my body language, and I add helpful gestures while minimizing distracting actions. | | | | | |
| 6. I pay attention to my speaking speed, and I attempt to speak slowly enough for learner comprehension and note-taking. | | | | | |
| 7. I am aware of my proxemic behaviors, and I try to distribute and maximize the time I spend facing different groups in the audience. | | | | | |
| 8. In small groups, I try to be aware of the social-consultive proxemic range. | | | | | |
| 9. I do not cling to the podium. | | | | | |
| 10. I minimize filler speech ("uh", "um", "ah", etc). | | | | | |
| 11. I stand up straight and keep my head up to make the most of my vocal timbre. | | | | | |
| **Total number of checkmarks per column:** | | | | | |

## Performance self-assessment score sheet

| | | | 1 | 2 | 3 | 4 | 5 |
|---|---|---|---|---|---|---|---|
| Assessment | Date | Scoring | | | | | |
| Sample | 23 July 2009 | # items with each score: | 1 × 1 | 3 × 2 | 3 × 3 | 3 × 4 | 1 × 5 |
| | | Value | 1 | 6 | 9 | 12 | 5 |
| | | Total score (sum of value line): 33 | | | | | |
| | | Percent success (divide score by maximum, 55): 60% | | | | | |
| 1 | | # items with each score: | ×1 | ×2 | ×3 | ×4 | ×5 |
| | | Value | | | | | |
| | | Total score (sum of value line): | | | | | |
| | | Percent success (divide score by maximum, 55): | | | | | |
| 2 | | # items with each score: | ×1 | ×2 | ×3 | ×4 | ×5 |
| | | Value | | | | | |
| | | Total score (sum of value line): | | | | | |
| | | Percent success (divide score by maximum, 55): | | | | | |

| Assessment | Date | Scoring | | | | | |
|---|---|---|---|---|---|---|---|
| 3 | | # items with each score: | ×1 | ×2 | ×3 | ×4 | ×5 |
| | | Value | | | | | |
| | | Total score (sum of value line): | | | | | |
| | | Percent success (divide score by maximum, 55): | | | | | |
| 4 | | # items with each score: | ×1 | ×2 | ×3 | ×4 | ×5 |
| | | Value | | | | | |
| | | Total score (sum of value line): | | | | | |
| | | Percent success (divide score by maximum, 55): | | | | | |
| 5 | | # items with each score: | ×1 | ×2 | ×3 | ×4 | ×5 |
| | | Value | | | | | |
| | | Total score (sum of value line): | | | | | |
| | | Percent success (divide score by maximum, 55): | | | | | |

# Measuring outcomes and ensuring success

## Chapter overview

As stated in Chapter 1, designing content "begins with the end in mind." The goal of medical education is to obtain maximum levels of learning. Chapter 4 discusses how to measure whether that endpoint has been met. Program evaluation is a hot topic in medical education these days, and this chapter analyzes not only the methods for measuring educational outcomes but also the results of applying these methods. The goal is to determine at a minimum whether learning has occurred, and, ideally, whether behavior has changed in response to an educational program.

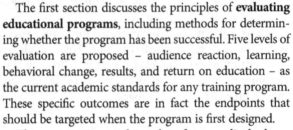

The first section discusses the principles of **evaluating educational programs**, including methods for determining whether the program has been successful. Five levels of evaluation are proposed – audience reaction, learning, behavioral change, results, and return on education – as the current academic standards for any training program. These specific outcomes are in fact the endpoints that should be targeted when the program is first designed.

The next section explains that, for a medical education program, **Level 1 success (audience reaction)** is the usual standard of evaluation and is quite rudimentary. Level 1 evaluation merely determines whether audiences liked the learning event, and thus is little more than a "smile sheet." Other Level 1 measurements can include simply counting the number of people who attended or asking learners whether they thought the education objectives were met.

The third section discusses how to document whether **Level 2 success** has occurred: namely, **learning**. It is surprising how infrequently this is done for medical education programs. One especially useful method for measuring success is with the use of audience response systems, employing pretest versus posttest results, with

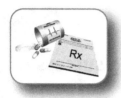

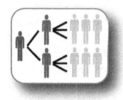

immediate feedback to both the instructor and the audience. Assessing learning not only can provide feedback to the learner but it can also show a measure of instructional effectiveness to the speaker, and, ultimately, evidence of success to the program organizers.

The fourth section presents various ways to measure, or measure by proxy, **Level 3 success (behavioral change)**. Ideally, a successful medical education initiative will lead to health care providers changing their habits in diagnosing, prescribing, or other practices. Available measures of Level 3 data suggest that medical education may be more successful when encouraging new behaviors than when discouraging previous behaviors, and that multiple exposures to the content may be much more beneficial for attaining educational success at Level 3.

The purpose of medical education – better care for patients – is discussed in the section on **Level 4 success (results)**. This outcome is rarely measured, and perhaps even more rarely achieved. Available data suggest that interactive medical education programs (instead of didactic lectures alone) may be best at reaching Level 4 success.

In medical education, the potential for **Level 5 success (return on education)** is huge, as discussed in the last section. This is analogous to the business concept of return on investment, except that the currency here is not money but rather the amount of health care being impacted by the resources required to implement a given educational program.

## Introduction

### Rationale and benefits

#### Does medical education "work"?

A debate is raging today in medical education: does it "work?" Certainly, students pass exams after taking a course, and specialists pass their boards after completing a residency, but it is now quite controversial as to whether this means that any given lecture or presentation really improves medical practice. It is not even clear how to measure whether it did.

Naysayers point to numerous academic studies showing that live meetings, written materials, and other ways of presenting new information to practitioners may not make any notable or sustained difference in how diagnoses are made, how patients are monitored, or whether evidence-based treatments or consensus treatment guidelines are applied in actual clinical practice (Tu and Davis, 2002;

Davis *et al.*, 1992, 1995, 1999; Fox and Bennett, 1998; Oxman *et al.*, 1995; Hodges *et al.*, 2001; Kroenke *et al.*, 2000; Sharma *et al.*, 2003; Davis, 2001). At the same time, other critics suggest that some educational programs, particularly continuing medical education (CME) sponsored by pharmaceutical and device companies, may work all too well, heavily influencing audience members to increase their use of sponsors' drugs and equipment while not necessarily improving best practice standards (Stahl, 2005; Wazana, 2000; Relman, 2001, 2003).

The real question may not be whether medical education "works" but how medical education can be designed, implemented, and evaluated to best facilitate learning, lead to transfer of knowledge into clinical practice, improve the skills of practitioners, and enhance the outcomes of patients.

## Outcomes: can you get there from here?

Documenting whether or not medical education programs change practitioner behavior may be difficult if the activities are designed to deliver a different outcome: namely, to follow a curriculum or to expose a large number of practitioners to the flood of new information that is constantly entering clinical medicine. This outcome is relatively easy to achieve. It should be no surprise, however, that educational activities designed only to expose practitioners to massive amounts of information may fail to change behavior.

Recently a consensus is emerging that modern medical education should strive to achieve something more ambitious: namely, making better practitioners and improving the health of their patients by providing educational activities for professionals that change their clinical behaviors and improve their skills in clinical practice (Mazmanian, 2005; Davis, 2006).

## Quantitative evaluation applied to medical education

Earlier chapters have discussed descriptive and qualitative aspects of assessing success and outcomes for individual components of educational events. The current state of the art is to go beyond this and measure whether educational presentations and events have quantitative impact and success.

For example, outcomes can address these questions:
- Did anyone learn anything?
- Did anyone who learned at the event retain that information later?
- Did the learning have an impact on medical practice in terms of helping the learner develop a new skill, make a diagnosis more accurately, or prescribe better treatment once the learner was back in the clinical practice setting?

These questions can be addressed with modern education methods, but measuring outcomes starts with the design of the program, not with the questions that follow a lecture. Thus, planning for organized assessments begins when an instructor starts to lay out content, bearing certain goals in mind. The results of those assessments can help identify strengths and weaknesses of a given lecture or presentation and allow continuous improvement in the performance and impact of a medical education program.

Realistically, it is time-consuming and difficult to measure learning. It is even more problematic to measure behavioral changes, because the methods for this are not well developed and many approaches are more intuitive than quantitatively validated. Most measurements of practice-based outcomes are simply too expensive to be practical. So what is a medical educator to do if educational outcomes are to be measured?

This chapter will demonstrate how an instructor can first identify several levels of goals for success in a medical education program and then structure measurements of that success. Examples will be given of methods used by medical educators as they have approached these same issues.

## Section 1

### Kirkpatrick's levels of evaluation

*If you don't know where you're going, any road will take you there.* (Lao Tze)

After giving a lecture, almost any instructor wants to know whether all the work of preparing and presenting the content was worth it. Donald Kirkpatrick (BioBox 4-1) is one of the pioneers of determining criteria to evaluate the success of an educational event or program. He has specifically established "Four Levels" of evaluation (Kirkpatrick and Kirkpatrick, 2006) (Figure 4-1). These include audience reaction (whether learners liked the program), learning (whether audiences understood the content and learned anything new), behavioral change (whether learners implement the specific information from that educational event in their practices), and results (whether patient care improves).

A fifth level of effectiveness has been proposed by Jack J. Phillips: return on education (Phillips, 2003) (Figure 4-2). For medical education, return on education

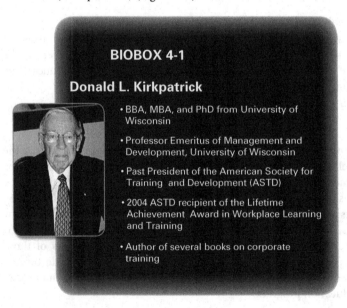

BIOBOX 4-1

**Donald L. Kirkpatrick**

- BBA, MBA, and PhD from University of Wisconsin

- Professor Emeritus of Management and Development, University of Wisconsin

- Past President of the American Society for Training and Development (ASTD)

- 2004 ASTD recipient of the Lifetime Achievement Award in Workplace Learning and Training

- Author of several books on corporate training

## Kirkpatrick's Four Levels of Evaluation

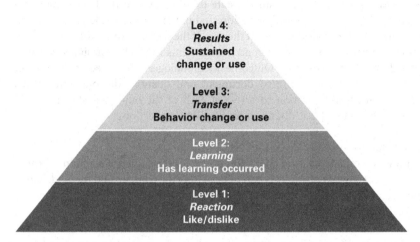

Figure 4-1. **Kirkpatrick's four levels of evaluation.** (Kirkpatrick and Kirkpatrick, 2006)

## Five Levels of Evaluating Success

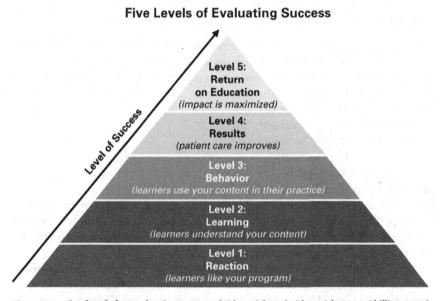

Figure 4-2. **Five levels for evaluating success.** (Kirkpatrick and Kirkpatrick, 2006; Phillips, 2003)

means maximizing the number of patients affected, or maximizing the effect on patients, per the effort, resources, time, and expense that the education program has invested in preparing and presenting the educational materials.

For a medical education instructor, knowing the goals of a program and how they will be measured is a key component of designing an education program in the first place. If the goal is only to be entertaining, one can casually survey the audience for people who are laughing or nodding off. If the goal is to meet objectives, the instructor can simply state the objectives at the beginning of the lecture, make sure each objective is addressed in the body of the lecture, and then summarize the objectives covered at the end. If the goal is to reach the higher levels on the Kirkpatrick pyramid, then additional items need to be designed within a medical education program. Outcome methodologies also need to be applied during and after the lecture to document and quantify the outcome results. Designing medical education to arrive at each of the outcomes shown for the five levels in Figure 4-2 is discussed in the following sections.

### Section summary: Kirkpatrick's levels of evaluation

Planning to evaluate medical education programs for audience reaction, learning, behavioral change, and results is part of designing the content, and methods can be employed to achieve the goal of documenting the quantitative outcome of any medical education activity.

## Section 2

### Level 1 success – reaction

For many years, the principal outcome measure of medical education has been the Level 1 evaluation, which looks at such aspects of the presentation as who attended the presentation, with the faulty assumption that events with large enrollments are successful. Level 1 evaluation also focuses on:

- How long did learners attend?
- Did learners like the speakers?
- Did learners like the handout?
- Did learners like the facility?
- Did learners like the topic?
- Did learners think that the program met the objectives?

Such evaluations, or "smile sheets," have many problems, including the fact that many participants do not complete them or turn them in, and those who do may represent a skewed population of participants who had the strongest reactions – not necessarily the typical reactions – to the activity.

Level 1 (Figure 4-1) (Kirkpatrick, 1994) is often evaluated by anecdotal methods that are hard to quantify, such as "positive buzz," verbal comments, or follow-up voicemail messages. Using audience response systems (see Chapter 1) can help with the collection of much more comprehensive data.

Some sample questions for measuring Level 1 success are given in Table 4-1.

### Section summary: Level 1 success – reaction

Evaluating whether audiences like a learning event is better than doing nothing, but it is essentially qualitative and impressionistic. Nevertheless, it can be helpful in

**TABLE 4-1:** Level 1 (reaction) evaluation questions for medical education

**The overall quality of the content was...**

| poor | subpar | fair | good | excellent |

**The organization of the content was...**

| poor | subpar | fair | good | excellent |

**The relevance of the content to my professional needs was...**

| poor | subpar | fair | good | excellent |

**Compared to a lecture, I enjoyed the workshop format...**

| much less | less | equal | more | much more |

**Based on my knowledge, the level of this activity was...**

| too basic | basic | appropriate | complex | too complex |

**The speaker's effectiveness at delivering the material was...**

| poor | subpar | fair | good | excellent |

performing a rudimentary program evaluation and can help guide future content development.

# Section 3

## Level 2 success – learning

The Level 2 evaluation involves assessing acquisition of new knowledge (Figure 4-2). Passing an exam after a presentation does not mean that learning has occurred. For example, Figure 4-3 shows that 73% of one Internet audience studied by the authors knew the right answer after participating in an online education program. However, without a baseline, this is not measuring learning. From the information in Figure 4-3, it is not even clear that this represents more knowledge than before the program, because it could also represent a decline in knowledge if the program included errors or was confusing. Thus, to show that learning has occurred, a baseline level of knowledge must be assessed. The best way to do this is a pretest of existing knowledge just prior to a program, often with automated (and anonymous) recording of group responses electronically via audience response keypads.

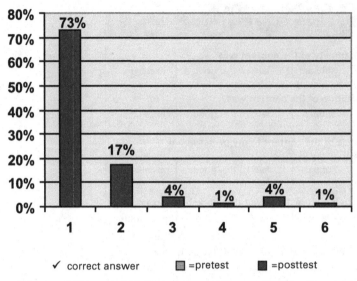

✓ correct answer        ▣ =pretest        ■ =posttest

**What would be your first-line preference for an ADHD patient with predominantly inattentive symptoms?**

✓ 1. Stimulant
   2. Atomoxetine
   3. Modafinil
   4. Guanfacine/clonidine

   5. Bupropion or other
      antidepressant
   6. Atypical antipsychotic

Figure 4-3 **Post-participation exam question for Internet online learning course.** Without a pre-course baseline, it is not clear whether this represents more knowledge than before the program. This is not measuring learning.

In principle, pretests are especially easy to apply to continuing medical education (CME) activities, because the current standard for planning a CME activity begins with a needs analysis that identifies gaps in knowledge of the targeted participants (Figure 4-4). However, some caution is warranted here because the audience members can only be aware of their own lack of knowledge in areas in which they are conscious of their incompetence (see Chapter 2 and Figure 2-13). Areas of ignorant bliss, where an audience member does not even know he or she does not know something (unconscious incompetence) will obviously not be assessed by this style of approach to needs assessment.

Nevertheless, pretest questions for participants should document whenever possible the lack of knowledge revealed via the needs analysis. Posttest questions should document whether learning occurred. To accomplish this, there is a definite art to writing audience response system (ARS) questions (see Chapter 1 and Table 1-5). For example, questions that show a high percentage of correct answers before an educational event has even started will prevent documentation of any learning on that issue due to a ceiling effect. Similarly, questions that are off the

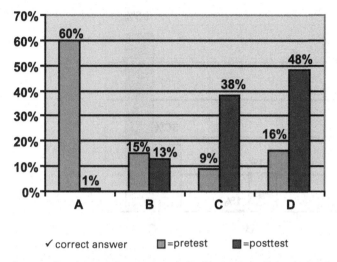

✓ correct answer        ■ =pretest        ■ =posttest

**Pretest: If a chart audit were conducted in your practice today, how many of your patients would have blood pressure, weight, and BMI recorded regularly?**

**Posttest: If a chart audit were conducted in your practice in one year, your goal would be to have what percentage of patients with blood pressure, weight, and BMI recorded regularly?**

A. Less than 10%                C. 50% or more (up to 75%)

B. 25% or more (up to 50%)      ✓ D. More than 75%

Figure 4-4. **Pretest and posttest exam question results.** Gaps in the knowledge of participants can show up if questions are asked before the presentation as well as after.

subjects being covered in the presentation, or that are too hard to understand even if relevant content is covered, risk having low percentages of correct answers not only before but also after the educational event.

An example of how learning can be documented is shown in Figure 4-5. A CME needs assessment had previously revealed that psychiatrists lacked understanding of metabolic issues affecting their patients who receive treatment with atypical antipsychotics. For this reason, the question shown in Figure 4-5 was posed to CME attendees. Indeed, this question documented that the audience did not know the correct answer prior to the lecture (pretest). Answers were scattered among correct and incorrect choices in the pretest. However, immediately following the lecture, the posttest showed that 95% of participants answered the question correctly. The audience members received this feedback on their improvement immediately as a pretest-to-posttest comparison. Thus, learning on this key point was documented for the audience, the instructor, and the CME program organizers. This is a good example of Level 2 evaluation of outcome (learning). As simple as this is, it is stunning how infrequently learning is ever measured or documented after a medical education event.

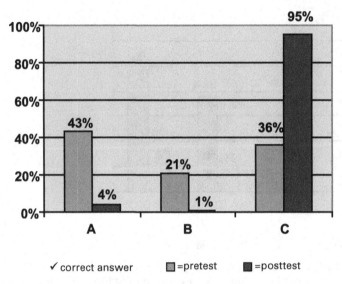

In patients who may develop metabolic problems, what is often the first change?

A. Weight gain                    ✓ C. Change in triglycerides

B. Fasting glucose levels greater
    than 100 mg/dl

Figure 4-5. **Sample Level 2 (learning) evaluation of medical education.** This figure shows results from 497 psychiatrists and other mental health care providers attending a Neuroscience Education Institute CME activity in New York City. The correct answer is C, change in triglycerides. Data were collected using audience response keypads for pretest (light gray) and posttest (dark gray). (Stahl *et al.*, 2006)

Documentation of learning has many important applications that can be used to modify and evaluate any medical education activity. Measurement of learning by evaluation of correct responses to factual questions in particular has many uses in the evaluation, design, and revision of medical education programs (Fox *et al.*, 1989; Prochaska and Velicer, 1997; Gagné, 1985; Brookfield, 1986). For example, if participants do not answer correctly following a lecture, the instructor can immediately go over this point and reinforce the correct answer. Sometimes an instructor is not aware of having confused the audience, and the number of correct responses can even go down following the lecture. Seeing this in the posttest allows the instructor to correct the audience misperception or his or her inadvertent misstatement. This can be done by the instructor immediately, prior to going on to other matters and leaving the audience confused or misinformed. Later, the content can be reevaluated to determine whether the answer was clear from the presentation. This is a type of formative test strategy and can be used not only to query the audience members but also to revise the content and the manner in which the instructor presents it in the future.

Also, sometimes most of the participants already know the answer to a pretest question (a not infrequent finding from pretest questioning, particularly if the questions are not skillfully composed or if the instructor was not expecting the audience to already know that information). When this occurs, the instructor can go through the material rapidly at the time of the presentation. After the presentation, the needs analysis can be updated if the question demonstrates that there is no longer an unmet need on this topic.

More likely, when participants already know the answer before the presentation, or when they do not improve their correct responses after hearing the presentation, the problem could very well be that the question needs to be rephrased.

An additional dimension to measurement of learning is its potential use in instructor evaluation. Measurement is especially useful for courses in which the same materials are presented by different instructors to similar audiences. At the beginning of a presentation, the instructor is aware from the pretest how much potential learning gain there is for a given audience. In the example of Figure 4-5, only 36% indicated the correct answer at the pretest. Thus, there was a potential learning gain on this point of 64%. Following the lecture, 95% answered the question correctly, so most of the potential learning was fulfilled. This should be the goal of each educational activity. Some instructors will be able to get better fulfillment of the potential learning gain than others. This is one way to evaluate and give feedback of teaching effectiveness to a faculty of instructors.

The goal is to write questions that document the expected knowledge gap before the lecture, then to present materials that effectively teach the information to fill this gap, and finally to document that this potential learning is largely fulfilled by each instructor.

Much can be done with skilled question writing, integrated with targeted content development and instructor preparation, combined with automated audience response keypad systems to document learning in medical education efforts. The minimum standard for medical education outcomes is to move from Level 1 outcomes to Level 2 (Figure 4-1) (Kirkpatrick, 1994) – namely, to document that learning has occurred.

## Learning versus mastery: long-term retention

Learning is linked to knowledge transfer not only as shown as a hierarchy by Kirkpatrick (Figure 4-1), but also by causative links (Figure 4-6). As stated repeatedly in this text, if the design of a medical education program begins with the end in mind, and if that end is to change behavior (far right in Figure 4-6), the learner will want to do more than just know the material. The learner will want to be confident in his or her mastery of this knowledge. According to Kirkpatrick (Kirkpatrick, 1994) and others (Fox et al., 1989; Prochaska and Velicer, 1997; Gagné, 1985; Brookfield, 1986), learning, mastery, and confidence are all precursors to transferring newly learned information into new skills or behavioral change (Level 3; discussed in the next section) (Figure 4-6). To be confident in material,

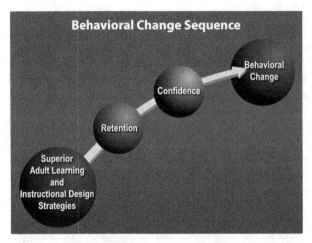

Figure 4-6. **Behavioral change sequence.** Kirkpatrick suggests that the precursor to behavioral change is confidence, and that the precursor of confidence is retention. (Kirkpatrick, 1994)

Kirkpatrick suggests that the learner must master it to a level of at least 70% correct answers and also retain this level of mastery at least until the information is applied later in the work setting.

Thus, learning is not enough. It is a necessary but not sufficient outcome from a medical education event. Not everyone who learns will change their behavior or improve their practice. On the other hand, it is difficult to conceive that participants would make changes in their clinical practice if they have not learned anything. Kirkpatrick suggests that the precursor to behavioral change is confidence, and that the precursor of confidence is retention (Figure 4-6). Retention is not just learning, but remembering it later. To document retention, learning must be measured after a delay. The "ladder of learning" suggests what different learning methods are expected to yield in terms of rates of retention 72 hours after an educational event (Chapter 1 and Figure 1-11).

The difference between retention and learning is also shown in Figure 4-7A and B. In this case, a program on bipolar disorder documented performance of the audience as only 52.2% correct answers on the pretest questions, but 86.9% correct answers on the posttest given on site immediately following the program (Figure 4-7A). The audience learned and learned well.

However, as shown in Figure 4-7B, retention was not nearly so high. Retention was measured in Figure 4-7B by conducting a mail survey of these same participants, who were queried on these same questions 6 weeks later. The content providing the answers was not mailed, only the test. The results were returned between 7 and 10 weeks following the course. This survey exemplifies one of the big problems with measuring retention by using survey methodology, since it is generally not possible to ensure a large follow-up population. This particular survey actually had a relatively high return rate for this method as many such surveys typically receive only around 3% return rates. However, here 15% of

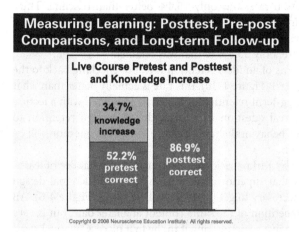

**Measuring Learning: Posttest, Pre-post Comparisons, and Long-term Follow-up**

**Live Course Pretest and Posttest and Knowledge Increase**

34.7% knowledge increase

52.2% pretest correct

86.9% posttest correct

**Figure 4-7A. Bipolar 1 pretest and posttest measurement of learning.** Performance of the audience is only 52.2% correct answers on the pretest questions but 86.9% correct answers on the posttest given on site immediately following the program.

**Measuring Learning: Posttest, Pre-post Comparisons, and Long-term Follow-up**

**Bipolar 1 Course Follow-up**
mailed at 6 weeks, returned 7-10 weeks after activity, return rate 15%

| % correct | change from pretest score (43.7%) | change from posttest score (87.1%) | % of increase retained* |
|---|---|---|---|
| 59.1% | 15.4% | -28.0% | 35.9% |

*For the average increase from pretest to posttest scores (43.4%), 35.9% of the increase was retained 7-10 weeks later.

**Figure 4-7B. Bipolar 1 follow-up measurement of learning.** Of the learning the participants showed on site immediately after the lecture, 35.9% of the increase was retained 7-10 weeks later.

participants returned a survey. This is nevertheless highly skewed to the population who responded, and there is no evidence that this subpopulation of responders represents the population who attended the course as a whole. In fact, it probably represents only the most motivated subpopulation.

The survey results showed that there was indeed measurable retention of information. Recall that these participants left the course knowing 86.9% of the correct answers. Seven to 10 weeks later, the score had dropped to only 59.1% correct answers. To measure retention, one must subtract what this audience knew before the course, namely, 52.2%. The change that persisted from the pretest to the posttest, that is, the retention rate, was only 15.4% better than baseline. Thus, audience members had dropped their posttest score by 28%. Another way of looking at these data is that, of the learning that the participants showed on site immediately after the lecture, only 35.9% of that was retained.

This may look bad in terms of an ideal retention rate, but checking back to the "ladder of learning" (Chapter 1, Figure 1-10), this rate is actually better than what others have reported for long-term retention of materials presented with a lecture and audiovisual aids. The real question is whether this is enough retention to inspire confidence and thus behavioral change (Figure 4-6). That question will be addressed in the next section.

The principles proposed by Kirkpatrick and illustrated by the "ladder of learning" (Figure 1-10) suggest that superior adult learning and instructional design strategies are going to be necessary to get high levels of retention (Figure 4-6). An old-fashioned strategy is repetition of the same content at a later date, but is very time inefficient compared to just remembering it in the first place. Chapter 1 dealt in detail with how to apply the principles of adult education to the design of medical education presentations that will lead to higher learning rates, higher retention rates, and thus confidence in the content. This is the necessary precursor of transferring that knowledge into clinical practice, arriving at Level 3.

### Section summary: Level 2 success – learning

Documentation of learning, especially through audience response systems, can provide feedback to the learner, a measure of instructional effectiveness to the speaker, and evidence of success to the program organizers.

## Section 4

### Level 3 success – behavior

Documentation of the outcomes of medical education programs now has the goal of going beyond mere documentation of learning. The current frontier is to show whether that learning passes into action and gets applied in clinical practice. Medical education is not about knowledge for knowledge's sake but about transfer from knowledge to practice – about learning that leads to performance improvement in clinical practice and skills development.

Documenting the attainment of Level 3 of Kirkpatrick's evaluation (Figure 4-1), however laudable, is much more easily said than done. In practice it is quite difficult to show that learning something about treatment, diagnosis, and laboratory testing gets transferred into clinical practice (Tu and Davis, 2002; Davis et al., 1992, 1995, 1999; Fox and Bennett, 1998; Oxman et al., 1995; Hodges et al., 2001; Kroenke et al., 2000; Sharma et al., 2003; Davis, 2001). Methods for measuring whether such transfer has occurred have many problems and limitations. Surveys (small number returned); focus groups (non-random and probably not representative samples); prescription audits (extremely expensive and structured for commercial applications, not for best-practices analyses); and chart audits

### Sample Proxy Level 3 (Behavior) Evaluation of Intent to Change After Medical Education

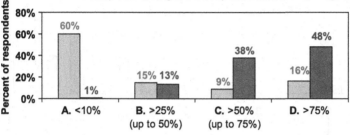

Figure 4-8. **Sample proxy Level 3 (behavior) evaluation of intent to change after medical education.** (Stahl *et al.*, 2006)

(expensive and confidentiality issues) are all examples of flawed methods that attempt to show that learning in CME can transfer into behavioral changes in practice (Tu and Davis, 2002; Davis *et al.*, 1992, 1995, 1999; Fox and Bennett, 1998; Oxman *et al.*, 1995; Hodges *et al.*, 2001; Kroenke *et al.*, 2000; Sharma *et al.*, 2003; Davis, 2001). It is not surprising that there is significant question as to whether transfer can be currently measured with affordable validated methods.

Rather than attempting to measure actual transfer of knowledge into clinical practice, a cheaper, easier, and more practical goal may be to show that the information in a medical education activity is theoretically applied. This theoretical behavioral application can be posed immediately after the instructional event, through an exercise that imitates clinical practice. "Imitation" Level 3 evaluations can be questions about attitudes, levels of confidence, intention to change clinical practice, or case studies. These outcome measurements are only proxies for what really happens in a clinical practice setting, but their facile measurement as part of the activity gives some quantification of whether the knowledge is being transferred, at least to model cases. This evaluation not only provides a measure of Level 3 success but also fulfills principles discussed elsewhere in this book. This evaluation:

- imitates "participating in a real situation" and "real-world experience/ application," the most active types of learning in the "ladder of learning"
- helps participants "emphasize future application."

A simple example of asking about intent to change behavior is shown in Figure 4-8. At best, such outcomes are merely proxies for what really happens in a clinical practice setting, yet these proxies can be measured as part of any

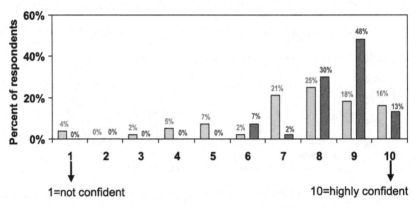

**Sample Proxy Level 3 (Behavior) Evaluation of
Confidence Level After Medical Education**

Please rate your level of confidence in using atypical antipsychotics
for the treatment of mania (pretest = light gray, **posttest = dark gray**)

Figure 4-9. **Sample proxy Level 3 (behavior) evaluation of confidence in prescribing after medical education.** (Arbor Scientia, 2007)

educational activity and at least show intent. Although not everyone who intends to change behavior will do so after the lecture, it is unlikely that those who do not intend to change behavior will do so. Thus, this can serve as a rudimentary estimate of the potential impact of the program, realizing that actual impact will probably be less.

Prior to hearing lectures on monitoring metabolic changes in psychiatry, the 297 participants at a Neuroscience Education Institute Psychopharmacology Academy in San Francisco in 2006 were asked how many of their patients currently have their blood pressures, weights, and body mass indices measured and recorded regularly. A very low number was indicated. After the lectures on monitoring metabolic status in psychiatry, the audience was asked how many patients they think should have these items measured and recorded regularly, and the results showed a huge shift upwards. Whether these participants will actually attain these goals is unknown, but this attitude shift would seem to be a necessary precursor to any actual behavior change.

A similar approach can be taken to measuring confidence by asking the audience members whether they are confident about an issue both before and after a lecture, looking for shifts towards more confidence. Even this yields a self-assessment opinion, not factual data based on learning. The study in Figure 4-9 assessed confidence levels in 56 psychiatric health care providers before and after an educational program on atypical antipsychotics, neurobiology, and diagnosis of related psychiatric disorders. Whether the participants would prescribe more

## Sample Proxy Level 3 (Behavior) Evaluation of
## Case Study Application After Medical Education

**Pretest (light gray):**
What would be your first-line preference for an
attention-deficit/hyperactivity disorder patient
with predominantly inattentive symptoms?

**Posttest (dark gray):**
A 20-year-old male who was briefly treated unsatisfactorily
for attention-deficit/hyperactivity disorder as a 10-year-old
is now struggling with his grades as a college sophomore.
He has attention deficit but not hyperactivity or impulsivity.
What would be your first choice for this patient?

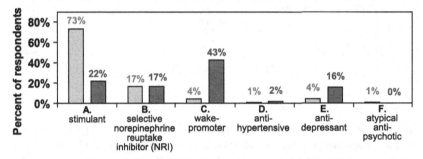

Figure 4-10. **Sample proxy Level 3 (behavior) evaluation of case study application after medical education.** (Stahl *et al.*, 2006)

atypical antipsychotics to manic patients is unknown, but the confidence shift documented here is a necessary precursor to any real behavioral change.

An example of the case-based approach to measuring behavioral change as an outcome of medical education is shown in Figure 4-10. This figure shows results from 297 psychiatrists and other mental health care providers attending a Neuroscience Education Institute CME activity in San Francisco. Data were collected using audience response keypads. Though there is no absolutely correct or incorrect answer, the results of the pretest agree with previous needs analyses (unpublished data from the Neuroscience Education Institute) showing that most practitioners greatly prefer stimulants for such patients. However, many psychiatrists are not willing to give stimulants to any adult and thus decline to treat attention-deficit/hyperactivity disorder (ADHD) in adults at all (pretest results, Figure 4-10).

To encourage more treatment of ADHD in adults, a CME activity was developed to outline off-label nonstimulant alternatives to treating inattentive symptoms. After the CME activity, participants were posed the case vignette to reassess audience preference of treatment for a patient with ADHD with predominantly inattentive symptoms. The posttest results (dark gray) document a shift away from stimulants to other alternatives.

True quantitative analyses of diagnosing or prescribing behaviors are rare because they are expensive and time-consuming to do. The rarity of Level 3

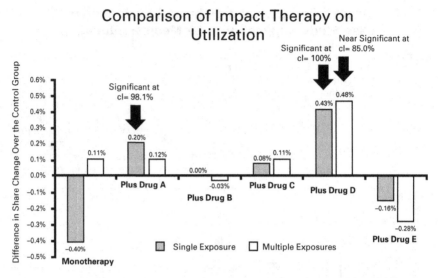

Figure 4-11. **A study in Level 3 (behavior) outcomes in prescription writing after medical education: single versus multiple exposures.** Changes in prescription-writing behaviors were analyzed in a test group of 1,184 physicians who attended CME programs, relative to a similar group of 2,109 control physicians. A main goal of the educational initiative was to encourage physicians' usage of appropriate augmentation therapies in order to achieve remission in depressed patients. Prescription data were collected for 6 months prior to first CME exposure and for 6 months after participation in the CME program. (Neuroscience Education Institute, 2004a)

quantitative assessments in medical education makes those that exist all the more valuable. Therefore, a few medical education programs with Level 3 assessments (and their implications) are presented here.

Figures 4-11, 4-12, and 4-13 show the quantitative measurement of medical education outcomes utilizing Level 3 assessments of changes in the prescription-writing behaviors of the physicians. Prescription audits were monitored for 6 months in physicians who attended the program and compared to prescription audits of matched physicians who did not attend the program.

Figures 4-11 and 4-12 are the results from the same study. Monotherapy with antidepressants for patients who were not in remission was targeted to be replaced by augmentation therapies, but not by any augmentation therapy. The objective of the program was to increase augmentation with drug A and drug D, but not with the others, and to do this at the expense of monotherapy. The program was a three-part series: first a half-day course, then a one-hour dinner meeting, followed by a one-hour teleconference.

This educational program also was designed to test whether multiple educational interventions were more effective than a single one. The results of the study showed directional changes in the targeted behaviors, namely, increases in augmentation

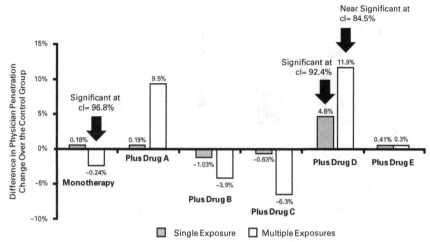

Figure 4-12. **Overall impact of education on physician penetration.** Physician penetration is defined as the ratio of the number of physicians using the therapy to physicians who participated in the CME. (Neuroscience Education Institute, 2004a)

with both drug A and drug D (Figure 4-11). Somewhat surprisingly, this figure also suggests that multiple interventions were no more effective than a single exposure to the materials. However, this was true only for the overall group (Figure 4-11), as Figure 4-12 suggests that the number of physicians who had the desired behaviors was greater if they attended multiple interventions than if they attended only one.

Although these results are preliminary and not definitive, they do suggest that when learning occurs (documented after the program with audience response keypad questions, not shown), one exposure to new material will lead physicians to do more frequently that which they are already doing (Figure 4-11), but it may take two or more exposures to new information to get physicians to start doing something they are not already doing (Figure 4-12).

A different educational program was designed to increase what was called desirable and rational drug combinations (rational polypharmacy) and to reduce costly, unproven, and undesirable drug combinations (questionable polypharmacy). The program emphasized evidence-based medicine and included realistic case scenarios. The Level 3 assessment measured changes in the prescription-writing behaviors of the 30 physicians who attended the CME event versus 30 matched controls, four months after the program. The results (Figure 4-13) show that physicians may be more likely to introduce new treatment practices (i.e. increase new augmentation strategies like rational polypharmacy) than to discontinue existing practices (i.e. decrease questionable polypharmacy) (Neuroscience Education Institute, 2004b). These findings are

## A Study in Level 3 (Behavior) Outcomes in Prescription Writing After Medical Education: New Versus Previous Behaviors

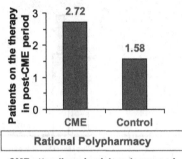

**Rational Polypharmacy**

CME-attending physicians increased
rational polypharmacy by 73%
over the control group,
significant at confidence level >99%

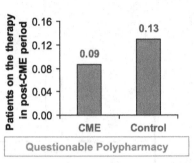

**Questionable Polypharmacy**

CME-attending physicians decreased
questionable polypharmacy by 23%,
but the difference is nonsignificant
at confidence level of 29%

Figure 4-13. **A study in Level 3 (behavior) outcomes in prescription writing after medical education: new versus previous behaviors.** Physicians may be more likely to introduce new treatment practices than to discontinue existing practices. (Neuroscience Education Institute, 2004b)

compatible with principles of adult learning discussed in Chapter 2 ("Draw on audience experience"): adults may have fixed habits and beliefs, so it may be easier for educational programs to get people to start a new behavior than to overcome old practices.

### Section summary: Level 3 success – behavior
Available Level 3 data suggest that medical education may be more successful when encouraging new behaviors than when discouraging previous behaviors and that multiple exposures may be beneficial for educational success. Documenting changes in physicians' behavior after medical education can be difficult, but proxy assessments can provide useful and more practical Level 3 assessments.

## Section 5

### Level 4 success – results

The ultimate goal for medical education is improvement in patient care – better quality of life, faster and more thorough recovery. Assessments of this goal are rare and sometimes impractical, but it may be very useful to design medical education content as if seeking this goal.

In one study of 17 formal didactic and/or interactive CME interventions (conferences, courses, rounds, meetings, symposia, lectures, and other formats),

**TABLE 4-2:** Characteristics of some CME programs that were successful at Level 4 (results for patients)

| | |
|---|---|
| **Attendees** | 83 pediatricians |
| **Topic** | Providing medication compliance strategies to patients with otitis media |
| **Program type** | 2.5-hour tutorial (didactic and discussion) plus educational materials, held twice |
| **Level 4 success** | At 6 months, significant improvement in proportion of patients with no missed doses |
| **Attendees** | 88 general internists and family physicians |
| **Topic** | Improving communication skills for 648 patients |
| **Program type** | Two 4-hour sessions with didactic presentation and interactive discussion; educational materials; practice with simulated patient; homework; role play |
| **Level 4 success** | At 3 months, significant reduction in patient distress score |
| **Attendees** | 74 pediatricians in community-based practices |
| **Topic** | Managing asthmatic patients |
| **Program type** | Two 2.5-hour seminars, 2 to 3 weeks apart; interactive video; small group discussion |
| **Level 4 success** | Up to 22 months, significant differences in health care outcomes as assessed by parent interviews about child health |

(Davis, 1999)

only five of the 17 assessed health care outcomes (Davis *et al.*, 1999). This study showed some evidence that interactive CME sessions – those that enhanced participant activity and provided the opportunity to practice skills – could change professional practice (Level 3 success, behavior) and sometimes could change health care outcomes (Level 4 success, results). Didactic lectures alone had no such efficacy. This is in accordance with the principles established in the "ladder of learning" (see Chapter 1, Figure 1-10) and Figure 4-1, Kirkpatrick's four levels of evaluation. Details about these successful programs are given in Table 4-2.

Modeling educational programs on these principles (geared toward Level 4 success) is particularly important because so many programs fail at Level 4. In another report of 12 studies of CME programs about hypertension control (Tu and Davis, 2002), only seven programs were successful at Level 3 (changing behavior) and none was effective at Level 4 (improving blood pressure levels of the patients).

Few programs are even evaluated at Level 4, so it is not clear how often medical education presentations clear this hurdle, but the data so far suggest that it might not be that often.

### Section summary: Level 4 success – results

The ultimate goal of medical education – better results for patients – is rarely achieved and certainly rarely documented. Interactive medical education programs may be best at reaching Level 4 success.

## Section 6

### Level 5 success – return on education

In medical education, the potential for return on the investment of time, effort, and resources is huge. Consider the situation presented in Figure 4-14. Medical educators who can positively impact the practices (Level 3 success) of an audience of six health care providers, each of whom then effectively treats three patients per week using information from that presentation (Level 4 success), would potentially improve the lives of 18 patients in that week alone. That is Level 5 success: one highly effective educational presentation can improve the lives of a great many

### Realm of Influence of Medical Education

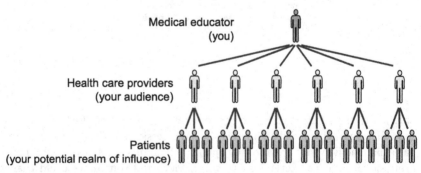

Figure 4-14. **Realm of influence of medical education.** The potential for return on educational investment can be exponential.

patients. Patient health and quality of life have immeasurable value. This is one of many reasons that working as a medical educator is so important.

### Section summary: Level 5 success – return on education

A multitude of patient lives can be affected by medical education; therefore, the potential for return on investment is huge, and so is the importance of a medical educator's work.

## Chapter summary

- Level 1 success (reaction) is when audience members enjoy an educational event; structured assessments can help document Level 1 success but are rather rudimentary and no longer state-of-the-art.
- Level 2 evaluations (learning) determine whether audience members understand the content; properly designed questions posed to an audience can guide learners and instructors alike to better instructional success.
- If a medical education presentation reaches Level 3 success (behavior change), that means that the audience members will change their practices in response to the teachings.
  - o True measures of Level 3 success can be expensive and/or difficult, but existing data suggest that
    - medical education may be more successful when encouraging new behaviors than when discouraging previous behaviors
    - multiple exposures may be beneficial for educational success.
  - o Proxy measures of Level 3 are often more practical and can include questions about attitudes, levels of confidence, intention to change clinical practice, or case studies.
- Level 4 success (results) means better patient care, which is infrequently measured and even less frequently achieved. Available data suggest that interactive educational sessions may be more likely than didactic lectures to improve health care outcomes.
- Level 5 success is return on education. Because medical educators can influence many health care providers, who then care for many patients, the potential for return on investment is extremely large.

## Progress check

Write down your answers in the pages provided in the back of the book or on a separate piece of paper so that you can re-take this test periodically without bias from your previous markings. Check your answers against the key in the back of the book and record your score in the ledger at the end of this quiz.
1. Of the following options, the best measure of Level 1 success is . . .
   a. Attendance counts
   b. Talking to participants to get verbal feedback

    c. Structured questions delivered via audience response systems

    d. Voluntary and anonymous open comment sheets left at every seat

2. The best measures of Level 2 success include all of the following *except*

    a. Pretest questions to measure baseline knowledge

    b. Posttest questions posed at the end of the session

    c. Questions focused on whether participants liked the session

    d. Immediate feedback provided to audiences about success

3. Which is Level 3 success? When audience members . . .

    a. Comprehend topics in your learning objectives

    b. Change their practices based on your information

    c. Like your presentation

    d. Remember your presentation for more than 6 months

4. Existing Level 3 evaluations suggest that all of the following are likely to be successful with medical educational programs, *except*

    a. Exposing audiences to educational topics twice

    b. Exposing audiences to educational topics three times

    c. Encouraging new favorable treatment practices

    d. Discouraging existing unfavorable treatment practices

5. All of the following are acceptable Level 3 evaluations, but which is the most difficult to execute?

    a. Questions about intent to change

    b. Presenting a case study patient to assess modeled treatment behavior

    c. Audits of prescribing practices

    d. Assessments of audience confidence in performing certain acts

6. Which of the following is Level 4 success?

    a. Results – patients exhibit improvement

    b. Results – physicians treat patients more effectively

    c. Behavior – patients act differently

    d. Behavior – physicians act differently

7. Available Level 4 evaluations of medical education programs suggest that only one of the following is true about improving patient outcomes. Which one?

    a. A majority of programs (more than half) are successful

    b. A majority of lectures (more than half) are successful

    c. Adding interactivity to learning might make programs more successful

    d. Improved care has been detected at more than 2 years after education

8. Which of the following is the best Level 5 success for medical education?

    a. Investing time in providing education, returning improved practices in physicians

    b. Investing money in providing education, returning improved practices in physicians

    c. Minimizing resources on providing education while maximizing number of physicians reached

    d. Investing time in providing education, returning improved patient care

## Performance ledger

| Assessment | Date | Scoring |
|---|---|---|
| 1 | | # correct answers: |
| | | percent correct answers (divide by 8): |
| 2 | | # correct answers: |
| | | percent correct answers (divide by 8): |
| 3 | | # correct answers: |
| | | percent correct answers (divide by 8): |
| 4 | | # correct answers: |
| | | percent correct answers (divide by 8): |
| 5 | | # correct answers: |
| | | percent correct answers (divide by 8): |

## Performance self-assessment

Photocopy this page or write down your answers on a separate piece of paper so that you can re-take this assessment periodically without bias from your previous markings. Record your score in the ledger on the next page.

| | 1 | 2 | 3 | 4 | 5 |
|---|---|---|---|---|---|
| | Poor, or Strongly Disagree | Fair, or Disagree | Average, or Neutral | Good, or Agree | Great, or Strongly Agree |
| **Level 1: Reaction** | | | | | |
| 1. I routinely administer structured Level 1 quizzes to assess whether learners like different aspects of my presentations. | | | | | |
| 2. I am open to changing and improving weaknesses or needs revealed in Level 1 assessments. | | | | | |
| 3. My Level 1 assessments routinely return good results or results that show improvement. | | | | | |

| Level 2: Learning | | | | | |
|---|---|---|---|---|---|
| 4. Before presentations, I routinely administer questions to measure baseline knowledge. | | | | | |
| 5. After presentations, I routinely administer questions to measure audience comprehension. | | | | | |
| 6. My audiences routinely show good improvement in learning from pretest to posttest. | | | | | |
| Level 3: Behavior | | | | | |
| 7. I routinely design content while considering principles likely to change physician behavior. | | | | | |
| 8. I regularly administer proxy assessments to examine whether audiences intend to change their behaviors because of my presentation. | | | | | |
| 9. Assessments usually indicate that my presentations will change the behaviors of my audiences. | | | | | |
| Level 4: Results | | | | | |
| 10. I routinely design my content with patient outcomes in mind. | | | | | |
| 11. I add interactivity to my educational initiatives, with the intention that it will improve patient outcomes. | | | | | |
| Total number of checkmarks per column: | | | | | |

## Performance self-assessment score sheet

| | | | 1 | 2 | 3 | 4 | 5 |
|---|---|---|---|---|---|---|---|
| Assessment | Date | Scoring | | | | | |
| Sample | 23 July 2009 | # items with each score: | 1×1 | 3×2 | 3×3 | 3×4 | 1×5 |
| | | Value | 1 | 6 | 9 | 12 | 5 |
| | | Total score (sum of value line): 33 | | | | | |
| | | Percent success (divide score by maximum, 55): 60% | | | | | |
| 1 | | # items with each score: | ×1 | ×2 | ×3 | ×4 | ×5 |
| | | Value | | | | | |

| Assessment | Date | Scoring | | | | | |
|---|---|---|---|---|---|---|---|
| | | Total score (sum of value line): | | | | | |
| | | Percent success (divide score by maximum, 55): | | | | | |
| 2 | | # items with each score: | ×1 | ×2 | ×3 | ×4 | ×5 |
| | | Value | | | | | |
| | | Total score (sum of value line): | | | | | |
| | | Percent success (divide score by maximum, 55): | | | | | |
| 3 | | # items with each score: | ×1 | ×2 | ×3 | ×4 | ×5 |
| | | Value | | | | | |
| | | Total score (sum of value line): | | | | | |
| | | Percent success (divide score by maximum, 55): | | | | | |
| 4 | | # items with each score: | ×1 | ×2 | ×3 | ×4 | ×5 |
| | | Value | | | | | |
| | | Total score (sum of value line): | | | | | |
| | | Percent success (divide score by maximum, 55): | | | | | |
| 5 | | # items with each score: | ×1 | ×2 | ×3 | ×4 | ×5 |
| | | Value | | | | | |
| | | Total score (sum of value line): | | | | | |
| | | Percent success (divide score by maximum, 55): | | | | | |

# Using interval learning in a comprehensive medical educational program

## Chapter overview

Chapter 5 introduces the "interval learning" concept, which can be employed to gain the most long-term benefit from the adult learning and psychology principles covered in previous chapters.

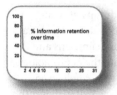

The first section discusses the shortcomings of "**bolus education**" approaches that are prevalent in classic medical education today. The loss of learned knowledge over time was quantified over 125 years ago in Hermann Ebbinghaus's "forgetting curve" and confirmed in more recent studies of medical education. Unfortunately, even the most effective learning methods don't break free of this forgetting curve.

The second section reveals how **interval learning** takes advantage of our understanding of the neurobiology of memory formation. The formation of stable memories requires three stages, which are called encoding, consolidation, and recall. *Encoding* of information happens during initial learning. *Consolidation* of memory requires the conversion of transient neuronal signals to lasting neurobiological changes such as neuronal growth, which occurs over days. These changes best occur under conditions that are free of interference from newly encoded information (e.g. during sleep). Periodic testing can stimulate the final *recall* stage of memory consolidation, thereby demonstrating that tests can be learning tools as much as assessment tools.

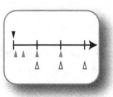

The third section covers how the Internet offers unique opportunities for **implementing interval education**, particularly in allowing busy learners flexibility in scheduling and locating their access to education. Healthcare providers can "learn by doing" by accessing their education at the point of care and putting their knowledge immediately into practice. If poorly

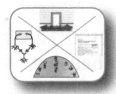

executed, however, online learning also carries the risk of fostering shallow, over-simplified understanding of complex information.

The final section demonstrates how a suite of novel content formats designed using adult education principles and delivered in "bite-sized" and repeated portions can provide a **comprehensive online education program**. The program utilizes lecture snippets, article quizzes, interactive case study drills, and mechanism of action videos to introduce the information. The learning interval is imposed via weekly self-assessment and learning tests. Based on the self-assessment tests, the program recommends content in the learner's weakest areas of knowledge and allows the learner to self-direct toward content based on the learner's newfound "conscious incompetence" in certain topics.

## Introduction

### Rationale and benefits

Medical education often presents new material as large data dumps at a single live event (e.g. a lecture or a symposium) not only because it is traditional, but also because this structure can be perceived as the most time-efficient for busy clinicians and their teachers. However, modern learning theory and new insights into the neurobiological basis of long-term memory formation show that the format of a single-event presentation of material is not very effective. Being presented with new material over time in bite-sized chunks and encountering the material again at a later time, particularly within a test, leads to more retention of information than does learning the same material as a large bolus in a single setting. This notion of learning over time, which is also called "interval learning" or "spaced learning," is particularly well suited to the Internet era. In this chapter, we describe how the concept of spaced learning can be combined with the adult education and psychology principles that we've discussed to provide effective learning of psychopharmacology over time in bite-sized and repeated portions. These bite-sized portions are presented in a variety of novel content formats that can be organized and structured as an "online fellowship" called the Master Psychopharmacology Program (www.neiglobal.com/mpptour). (see Stahl *et al.*, 2010).

## Section 1

### Bolus education: easy to forget

Classic medical education clings to the perception that learning happens in a single instance; this is why most new information is dispersed via live programs with a bolus of material covered with the once-over-easy approach. However, research shows that this approach may be one of the best ways to *forget* information.

## The forgetting curve

Over 125 years ago, Hermann Ebbinghaus established the "forgetting curve" (Figure 5-1). With this simple concept, he demonstrated that over time, there is a dramatic loss in the retention of new material learned in a single session. Since Ebbinghaus's time, a voluminous amount of research has confirmed this simple but important fact: the retention of new information degrades rapidly unless it is reviewed in some manner. A modern example of this loss of knowledge without repetition is a study of cardiopulmonary resuscitation (CPR) skills that demonstrated rapid decay in the year following training. By 3 years post-training, only 2.4% were able to perform CPR successfully (McKenna and Glendon, 1985). Another recent study of physicians taking a tutorial that they rated as very good or excellent showed a mean increase in knowledge scores from 50% before the tutorial to 76% immediately afterward. However, score gains were only half as great 3 to 8 days later, and there was no significant knowledge retention measurable at all at 55 days (Bell *et al.*, 2008). Similar results from follow-up studies of knowledge retention from continuing medical education programs were shown in Chapter 4, Section 3.

## Improving bolus education: tastier, but still missing the key ingredient

In Chapter 1, Section 9, we discussed higher-impact learning formats, and in particular the ladder of learning (Figure 1-10). Recall that the top rungs of learning

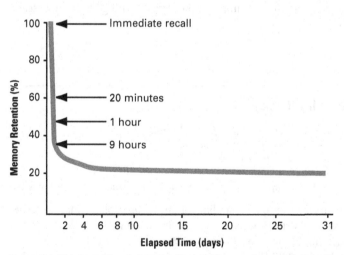

**The Forgetting Curve**

Figure 5-1. **The forgetting curve.** The "forgetting curve" was developed by Hermann Ebbinghaus in 1885. Ebbinghaus memorized a series of nonsense syllables and then tested his memory of them at various periods ranging from 20 minutes to 31 days. This simple but landmark research project was the first to demonstrate that there is an exponential loss of memory unless information is reinforced.

included the "immediate use of learning" and "practice by doing," which are techniques that are difficult to use in the traditional learning format.

### On-demand education

A popular current notion for improving the retention of newly presented medical information and subsequently effecting confidence and behavioral change (discussed in Chapter 4, Figure 4-6) is to depart from the classroom or the conference center and take the teaching closer to the point of delivery of medical care (Curran and Fleet, 2005). The idea here is that the effectiveness of traditional clinical education, especially continuing medical education, is limited because the clinician does not choose the topic, the pace of the program, or the place of the learning and cannot get the material when and where it is really needed – namely, at the point of care (POC). If healthcare providers could access the right information at the right time to satisfy questions that arise from clinical practice (at the POC), they could apply top-rung learning strategies to their learning and immediately improve medical care and patient outcomes. However, even this approach fails to recognize that information learned and used at the POC is likely to be forgotten if it is not repeated at a later time. Fortunately, various ways to repeat the information over time are available and can improve the transfer of new information into clinical practice as stable new behaviors.

### Section summary

Bolus education is not effective in producing long-term knowledge retention because there is a rapid loss of knowledge after a single introduction to material. More effective learning methods can improve the initial learning but cannot escape the knowledge loss.

## Section 2

### Interval learning: play it again

> *You can get a good deal from rehearsal,*
> *If it just has the proper dispersal.*
> *You would just be an ass,*
> *To do it en masse,*
> *Your remembering would turn out much worsal.*        – Neisser's Law

Recent advancements in our understanding of the neurobiology that underlies normal human memory formation have revealed that learning is not an event, but rather a process that unfolds over time (Sisti *et al.*, 2007; Lee, 2009; O'Neill *et al.*, 2010; Squire *et al.*, 2003; Fields, 2005). Thus, it is not surprising that learning strategies that repeat information over time enhance its retention (Fields, 2005; Glenberg and Lehman, 1980; Toppino *et al.*, 1991; Landauer and Bjork, 1978; Karpicke and Roediger, 2008; Storm, 2010; Pashler *et al.*, 2007). Although almost any type of review increases retention, the objective is to structure the repetition of exposure to materials in a manner that is time efficient and relevant and links new knowledge to old knowledge, engages the learner, offers feedback on the accuracy of information recalled, and allows self-directed selection of which material to repeat (preferably, only that which has been already successfully encoded into memory).

Given that clinicians face an ever-expanding body of knowledge and yet have less and less time in which to learn, busy practitioners who wish to upgrade their skills and transfer new information into their clinical practice would greatly benefit from learning paradigms that adopt *more efficient* learning and retention strategies. The goal is to spend less *overall* time on both learning (encoding) *and* retaining (consolidating) new material despite the extra time required for repetition in order to retain the information. When this goal is achieved, it should also result in more *effective* recall so that new information is transferred into clinical practice (Figure 4-6).

## Don't fight your neurobiology

Why do we forget? We forget because memory is malleable. The establishment of stable memories is not a single process; instead, it is composed of three stages of neurobiological processing (Figure 5-2): encoding, consolidation, and recall (Lee, 2009; O'Neill *et al.*, 2010; Squire *et al.*, 2003). Encoding may occur in one part of the brain (hippocampus) and exist primarily as transient electrical and chemical events.

However, the neurobiological processes of encoding have a limited shelf life, and these memories must be stabilized or "consolidated" by transferring them into other brain areas, such as the cortex. These transient electrical and chemical events must be converted over the course of days into longer-lasting neurobiological processes that involve structural neuronal changes, synapse formation or remodeling, and even the creation of new neurons (Sisti *et al.*, 2007; Lee, 2009; O'Neill *et al.*, 2010; Squire *et al.*, 2003; Fields, 2005; Stahl, 2010; Sweatt, 2009).

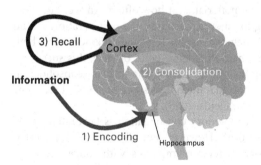

Figure 5-2. **The stages of learning.** (1) Information is encoded into the hippocampus for short-term storage. (2) Consolidation begins the process of forming long-term memory by transferring transient hippocampal neuronal signals to the cortex. (3) Recall and interval learning begin to reinforce the creation of neuronal pathways in the cortex for long-term storage of information.

Initially, new memories in the encoding and early consolidation stages are unstable and vulnerable to degradation by interference from ongoing experiences; eventually, however, they can become long-lasting (Sisti *et al.*, 2007; Lee, 2009; O'Neill *et al.*, 2010; Squire *et al.*, 2003; Fields, 2005). However, even long-term memories are not necessarily fixed and stable. A process known as "reconsolidation" allows an old memory to be recalled and updated (Lee, 2009; O'Neill *et al.*, 2010). That is a good thing because it allows a physician to modify his or her behavior; for example, he or she might change prescribing decisions based on new diagnostic criteria or a recently discovered side effect. Reconsolidation presents the opportunity to not only retrieve a stable memory, but also modify it, and in so doing, update clinical skills and behaviors.

### Sleep on it
New memories and experiences interfere with the conversion of recently encoded information into stable memories. Transferring memory from the encoding stage, which occurs during alert wakefulness, into consolidation must occur when interference from ongoing new memory formation is reduced (Lee, 2009; O'Neill *et al.*, 2010). These conditions are satisfied during sleep, especially non-rapid eye movement sleep, when the hippocampus can communicate with other brain areas without interference from new inputs (Strickgold *et al.*, 2001; Marshall and Born, 2007; Maquet, 2001).

Interestingly, memory can also be transferred from encoding into consolidation during offline periods while awake (Lee, 2009; O'Neill *et al.*, 2010). The essential concept for consolidation and thus storage of memory is that the waking neuronal activity that occurred during encoding must be reactivated by repetition (i.e. "replayed"), while either awake or asleep, with the same firing patterns associated with the initial learning.

### When should you hit the replay button?
When should the learner replay the material, and how often? Answers to these questions are only now beginning to emerge. Certainly, the first iteration should employ all the best educational strategies available to encode memory for a high degree of immediate recall. From a neurobiological point of view, this successful encoding, followed by a good sleep the night after, sets the stage for consolidation into long-term memory but does not guarantee it (Sisti *et al.*, 2007; Lee, 2009; O'Neill *et al.*, 2010; Squire *et al.*, 2003; Fields, 2005).

Numerous studies now show that memory consolidation is facilitated by re-iterating the material spaced over time. However, not all intervals are created equal. As a general rule, memory formation improves with longer intervals between reiteration of information, but only up to a point. That is, repetition right after the initial presentation, such as in sequential lectures in a symposium, is not as effective as repeating that same information days (but not months) later. This improvement in memory formation versus bolus education can be called the "spacing effect" (Bell *et al.*, 2008; Curran and Fleet, 2005; Fields, 2005; Glenberg and Lehman, 1980; Toppino*et al.*, 1991; Landauer and Bjork, 1978; Karpicke and

Roediger, 2008; Storm *et al.*, 2010; Pashler *et al.*, 2007; Roediger and Karpicke, 2005; Johnson and Kiviniemi, 2009; Cook *et al.*, 2006).

However, one exception to the spacing effect advantage is when providing feedback to the learner. Feedback is a form of repetition that is most effective when given immediately after a learning experience, especially when learning facts and particularly after a learner has made an error that needs correction (Pashler *et al.*, 2007; Cook *et al.*, 2006).

### Déjà vu all over again?
Does repetition mean that the student should just review the same material over and over? It turns out that the forgetting rate for information is determined not only by the intervals between repetitions, but also by the type of reiteration. For example, simple restudying allows the learner to reexperience all of the material but actually produces poor long-term retention (Storm *et al.*, 2010; Pashler *et al.*, 2007; Roediger and Karpicke, 2005). Restudying is commonly used in learning environments because it is often the learner's only option and because it apparently leads to mastery of the information in the short term. However, studies using delayed testing show that this mastery does not translate into long-term knowledge.

### Interval learning through tests
Is testing an assessment tool or a learning strategy? The answer is both. Tests not only assess knowledge, but also engage the third stage of memory formation: the recall stage. To the surprise of many, tests have proven to be very positive and productive ways to reinforce learning and increase long-term retention. In fact, the best way to retain new information may be to review it until it is encoded (i.e. can be recalled correctly in an immediate posttest), and then to be tested on it in successive intervals of first a few days to a week, then again in a week or two (Figure 5-3). This method, known as "expanded retrieval," has resulted in greater long-term retention versus mere iterative review of materials (Karpicke, 2008; Storm *et al.*, 2010; Pashler *et al.*, 2007; Roediger and Karpicke, 2005; Johnson and Kiviniemi, 2009; Cook *et al.*, 2006).

Expanded retrieval can be contrasted with "uniform retrieval," in which the intervals between successive tests are the same. Uniform retrieval is beneficial in cases in which the initial encoding of information was inaccurate or incomplete. However, as long as information was properly encoded, the expanded retrieval

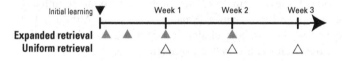

Test administration time points

Figure 5-3. **Expanded retrieval versus uniform retrieval.** Expanded retrieval testing intervals lead to better long-term retention of information. Uniform retrieval is beneficial for correcting encoding errors.

method is more effective because the increasing interval between tests requires greater effort in the recall stage, and this effort seems to promote long-term retention (Karpicke and Roediger, 2008). Expanded retrieval shows particular advantage with knowledge that is vulnerable to loss, such as information that was encoded concurrently with similar information that could interfere with its recall. Now the question is: how do you incorporate expanded retrieval into an educational program?

### Section 2 summary

Interval learning facilitates the transfer of long-term memory by stimulating the consolidation and recall stages of memory formation. Interval learning also allows the critical long-term memory-forming neurobiological processes that occur during sleep to play their part. Tests engage the recall stage of learning, and using expanded retrieval spacing can enhance long-term memory formation.

## Section 3

### The Internet: a web of learning or a tangled web?

As the vehicle for the delivery of well-designed medical education, the Internet provides many advantages, including the facilitation of encoding, consolidation, and recall of information. Because e-learning is on demand, it accommodates the busy clinician's schedule and enables the learner to review information in multiple places, including at the POC, and at multiple times until it can be recalled (Bell *et al.*, 2008; Curran and Fleet, 2005; Johnson and Kiviniemi, 2009; Cook *et al.*, 2006; Kerfoot, 2008, 2009; Kerfoot and Bortschi, 2009). Webcasts and lectures can be recorded and replayed at the learner's convenience. Immediate feedback on tests taken with the initial presentation of materials can be provided to correct encoding errors (Pashler *et al.*, 2007; Cook *et al.*, 2006).

Thereafter, e-learning platforms can automatically invite users back for review or testing according to their expanded retrieval regimen (Karpicke and Roediger, 2008). Even smartphones can provide an additional access point for scheduled online quizzes. Studies of online spaced medical education programs show that such programs can lead to more long-term retention of information than single-event-based learning activities, although the improvement can be modest.

Web-based teaching, however, can have the problem of poor compliance, especially with follow-up testing activities (Small *et al.*, 2009). Although tests may be more effective than review, busy clinicians may avoid them because they take more effort and their value is not well appreciated.

Furthermore, critics point out that the Internet is an environment that promotes cursory reading, hurried and distracted thinking, and superficial learning (Small *et al.*, 2009). Even as the Internet grants us easy access to vast amounts of information, it may be turning us into shallow thinkers who are incapable of critical reflection and deliberation.

It is thus important that e-learning programs avoid creating a false aura of exactness by reducing medical problems to a form that is amenable to objective measurement. Programs need to leave room for the art of medicine because every case differs from all others; the learner also needs to develop an eye for nuance, context, and ambiguity (Small *et al.*, 2009).

### Section 3 summary
The Internet can offer great learning advantages because its flexibility is amenable to addressing all three phases of learning through expanded retrieval techniques. However, compliance may be poor, and programs must be carefully designed to avoid oversimplification of the information.

## Section 4

### The Master Psychopharmacology Program (MPP)

#### Overview
The Master Psychopharmacology Program (MPP) is an online presentation of the topics in psychopharmacology that is designed to teach information such that it will be transferred into clinical practice. It employs the principles of adult learning to maximize the encoding of new information and follows up with expanded retrieval techniques in various formats, including tests (Figure 5-4). Specifically, original presentations of content are designed to be delivered in multiple novel online formats (Figures 5-5 to 5-8; Tables 5-1 and 5-2), to be bite-sized, to take only minutes to complete rather than an hour, and to require interactivity every minute. Moreover, online testing is extensively integrated into the MPP as both an assessment tool and a learning tool during reiterations of material. Finally, numerous supplementary activities are made available for self-directed learning so that participants can choose additional sources of information to either help them encode difficult-to-learn material or provide them with additional opportunities to consolidate easier topics in other formats and upon demand (see Stahl *et al.*, 2010).

### Novel content formats

What is different about the online educational program of the MPP is that psychopharmacology content is also presented in various novel formats as bite-sized multiples, grouped together into an "online fellowship" with a new activity link e-mailed every week (Figures 5-4 to 5-8; Tables 5-1 and 5-2). The MPP encourages participants to complete all of the activities, one per week, by investing about 10–20 minutes each week for at least 6 months. Once a month, there is a short lecture, which is called a "snippet" (Figure 5-5); a relevant article selected from the literature with pre- and posttesting (Figure 5-6); a new mechanism of action (MOA) lesson that is an animation with narration (Figure 5-7); and a case study, which is called a "drill" (Figure 5-8). Tests are embedded into each of these four formats.

# Overview of the Master Psychopharmacology Program

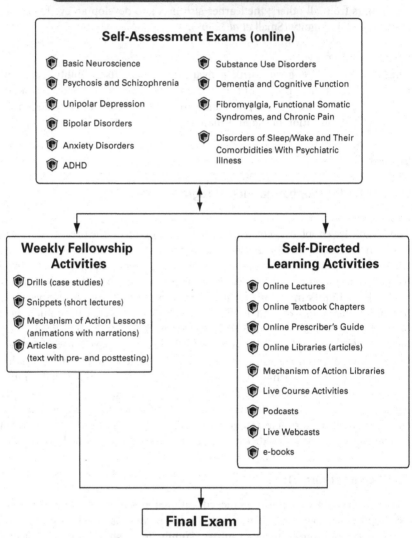

**Master Psychopharmacology Program (online)**

## Self-Assessment Exams (online)

- Basic Neuroscience
- Psychosis and Schizophrenia
- Unipolar Depression
- Bipolar Disorders
- Anxiety Disorders
- ADHD
- Substance Use Disorders
- Dementia and Cognitive Function
- Fibromyalgia, Functional Somatic Syndromes, and Chronic Pain
- Disorders of Sleep/Wake and Their Comorbidities With Psychiatric Illness

## Weekly Fellowship Activities

- Drills (case studies)
- Snippets (short lectures)
- Mechanism of Action Lessons (animations with narrations)
- Articles (text with pre- and posttesting)

## Self-Directed Learning Activities

- Online Lectures
- Online Textbook Chapters
- Online Prescriber's Guide
- Online Libraries (articles)
- Mechanism of Action Libraries
- Live Course Activities
- Podcasts
- Live Webcasts
- e-books

## Final Exam

Figure 5-4. **Overview of the Master Psychopharmacology Program.** The Master Psychopharmacology Program includes self-assessment exams on 10 subtopics in the field that identify subject areas requiring further study. Numerous self-directed learning activities are provided to master that material. Simultaneously, the participant completes 24 fellowship activities, which are emailed weekly in one of four formats: a case study, a short lecture, a mechanism of action animation, or an article. Finally, after completing self-directed learning activities and the 24 fellowship activities, the participant takes a final exam to receive a certificate of completion and become designated as a Master Psychopharmacologist.

## Snippet

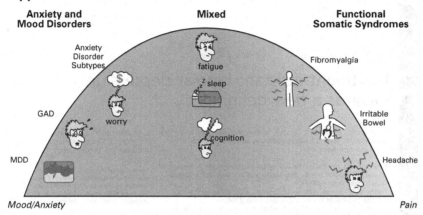

GAD=generalized anxiety disorder; MDD=major depressive disorder

Figure 5-5. **Snippet.** Once a month, the MPP provides a short lecture, called a Snippet, which is up to 15 minutes in length, with a pretest and a posttest question. Shown here is a screen shot of one of the slides from a snippet; the slide is seen while the lecturer is heard explaining the content.

The MPP is currently structured so that new content is presented weekly in a novel format; the participant is encouraged toward self-directed review via access to archived fellowship activities as well as additional online materials (Figures 5-4 to 5-8, Table 5-1). Self-direction allows flexibility for the participant to choose additional materials based on his needs. He may choose materials that help him encode particularly difficult new content, or he may wish to consolidate already encoded information by repetition so that the knowledge will transfer into clinical practice.

In contrast, interval learning theory might suggest rigidly programming reiterations of new material in these four different formats (Figures 5-4 to 5-8) over consecutive weeks. Other studies suggest, however, that spaced learning is not always better than massed/bolus learning (Son, 2010), particularly when the information has not been encoded properly in the first place. In these instances, participants will choose to mass their study until they have adequately learned the material. This learner's choice has also shown advantages over forced spacing in encoding and consolidating information.

Thus, the MPP promotes better learning by adapting the best educational design to facilitate the encoding of new materials through engaging, novel, and bite-sized presentations of new material. The participants are allowed the flexibility to either mass their study or space their learning, depending on their needs (albeit with some testing as forced spacing to receive full credit and ensure progress toward completion).

## Snippets

Although live lectures are usually 60 minutes in length, online viewers rarely watch a 1-hour lecture from beginning to end. Many will stay logged on to an online

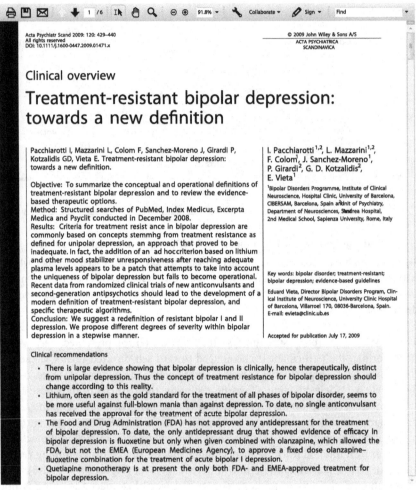

Acta Psychiatr Scand 2009: 120: 429–440
All rights reserved
DOI: 10.1111/j.1600-0447.2009.01471.x

ACTA PSYCHIATRICA
SCANDINAVICA

Clinical overview

# Treatment-resistant bipolar depression: towards a new definition

Pacchiarotti I, Mazzarini L, Colom F, Sanchez-Moreno J, Girardi P, Kotzalidis GD, Vieta E. Treatment-resistant bipolar depression: towards a new definition.

**Objective:** To summarize the conceptual and operational definitions of treatment-resistant bipolar depression and to review the evidence-based therapeutic options.
**Method:** Structured searches of PubMed, Index Medicus, Excerpta Medica and Psyclit conducted in December 2008.
**Results:** Criteria for treatment resistance in bipolar depression are commonly based on concepts stemming from treatment resistance as defined for unipolar depression, an approach that proved to be inadequate. In fact, the addition of an ad hoc criterion based on lithium and other mood stabilizer unresponsiveness after reaching adequate plasma levels appears to be a patch that attempts to take into account the uniqueness of bipolar depression but fails to become operational. Recent data from randomized clinical trials of new anticonvulsants and second-generation antipsychotics should lead to the development of a modern definition of treatment-resistant bipolar depression, and specific therapeutic algorithms.
**Conclusion:** We suggest a redefinition of resistant bipolar I and II depression. We propose different degrees of severity within bipolar depression in a stepwise manner.

I. Pacchiarotti[1,2], L. Mazzarini[1,2], F. Colom[1], J. Sanchez-Moreno[1], P. Girardi[2], G. D. Kotzalidis[2], E. Vieta[1]

[1]Bipolar Disorders Programme, Institute of Clinical Neuroscience, Hospital Clinic, University of Barcelona, CIBERSAM, Barcelona, Spain and[2]Unit of Psychiatry, Department of Neurosciences, Sant'Andrea Hospital, 2nd Medical School, Sapienza University, Rome, Italy

Key words: bipolar disorder; treatment-resistant; bipolar depression; evidence-based guidelines

Eduard Vieta, Director Bipolar Disorders Program, Clinical Institute of Neuroscience, University Clinic Hospital of Barcelona, Villarroel 170, 08036-Barcelona, Spain.
E-mail: evieta@clinic.ub.es

Accepted for publication July 17, 2009

**Clinical recommendations**

- There is large evidence showing that bipolar depression is clinically, hence therapeutically, distinct from unipolar depression. Thus the concept of treatment resistance for bipolar depression should change according to this reality.
- Lithium, often seen as the gold standard for the treatment of all phases of bipolar disorder, seems to be more useful against full-blown mania than against depression. To date, no single anticonvulsant has received the approval for the treatment of acute bipolar depression.
- The Food and Drug Administration (FDA) has not approved any antidepressant for the treatment of bipolar depression. To date, the only antidepressant drug that showed evidence of efficacy in bipolar depression is fluoxetine but only when given combined with olanzapine, which allowed the FDA, but not the EMEA (European Medicines Agency), to approve a fixed dose olanzapine–fluoxetine combination for the treatment of acute bipolar I depression.
- Quetiapine monotherapy is at present the only both FDA- and EMEA-approved treatment for bipolar depression.

Figure 5-6. **Article.** Once a month, the MPP provides an article in text form with a pretest and a posttest question. Shown here is a screen shot of one of the journal articles.

educational activity for only several minutes. One solution is to shorten the lecture to a "snippet" of fewer than 15 minutes (Figures 5-4 and 5-5; Table 5-1). Indeed, as the MPP has shortened the length of lectures, there have been increases in both the number of snippets viewed in their entireties and the total amount of time logged on to the program. It appears that for viewer engagement in online activities in general and lectures in particular, less is more.

In order to integrate the snippets into the MPP, each lecture begins with a pretest question about the content. After the viewer chooses an answer, the lecture begins. Posttests are designed to be taken after viewing the snippet. Answers do not have to be correct, but the viewer must complete the test to receive credit toward completing the online fellowship.

## Mechanism of Action Lesson

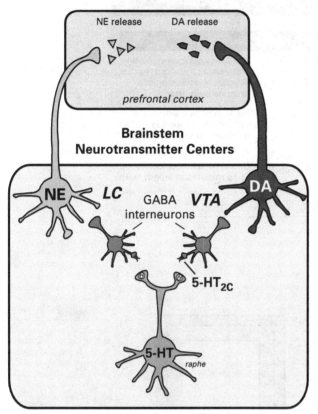

GABA=γ-aminobutyric acid; NE-norepinephrine; DA=dopamine; LC=locus coeruleus; VTA= ventral tegmental area; 5-HT=serotonin

Figure 5-7. **Mechanism of action lesson.** Once a month, the MPP provides an animation with narration of a mechanism of action concept from psychopharmacology. This explains either a disease action or a drug action, with a pretest and a posttest question. Shown here is a screen shot of one of the animations of a mechanism of action lesson; the animation is seen while a narrator is heard explaining the content.

### Articles

Text material is made available from either the published literature or newsletters that are specifically written for the MPP (Figures 5-4 and 5-6; Table 5-1). Articles begin with a pretest and end with a posttest, both of which must be completed to receive credit. Original articles with highly technical methods and jargon are not popular; after reading these articles' abstracts and possibly the beginning of their discussions, many viewers either skip these articles entirely or jump to the end to

**TABLE 5-1:** Fellowship Activities of the Master Psychopharmacology Program

| Name of Activity | Type of Activity | Description |
| --- | --- | --- |
| **Drill** | Case Study | Interactive exercise evaluating and treating a real case from a psychopharmacologist's practice over time |
| **MOA** | Animation | Flash animation with narration of a visually compelling disease mechanism or drug action |
| **Article** | Text | Article from the literature |
| **Snippet** | Short Lecture | Section of a longer lecture, up to 15 minutes in length, with slides |

MOA=mechanism of action

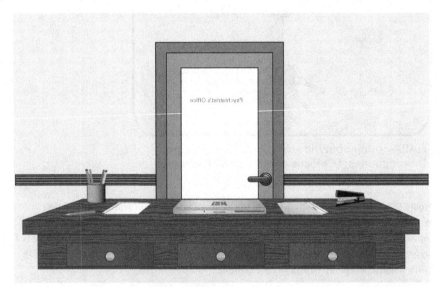

Figure 5-8. **Drill.** Once a month, the MPP provides an interactive case study, called a Drill. This lesson provides the viewer with an opportunity to "look over the shoulder" of a senior psychopharmacologist to see how s(he) handles complex clinical issues such as treatment resistance, treatment intolerance, multiple medications, the integration of psychotherapy, and comorbidities, with multiple previous examiners and prescribers. Shown here is a screen shot of the beginning of the case, which is followed over time with iterative trial-and-error prescribing of new treatments or new combinations and with outcomes (good or bad) over several months of treatment.

**TABLE 5-2**: Self-Assessment Exam: Attention-Deficit/ Hyperactivity Disorder (ADHD)

Your colleague asks you for advice on how to treat an ADHD patient with severe liver damage caused by many years of heavy drinking. You know that while most medications used for ADHD should be used with caution or not at all in patients with cardiac impairments, there is only one drug that requires special care when prescribing it to a person with liver impairment. Which drug is it?

| Answer Choices | Peer Answers | Your Answer |
|---|---|---|
| A. lisdexamfetamine | 15% | |
| B. d-methylphenidate | 2% | |
| C. d,l-methylphenidate | 2% | |
| D. atomoxetine | 78% | X |
| E. d,l-amphetamine | 1% | |
| F. d-amphetamine | 3% | |

The MPP divides the field into 10 areas, and the Self-Assessment Exams ask 10-15 questions in each area, with the correct answers given as soon as the learner answers them. The learner is shown how others have answered each question and is given explanations of each answer. The test is thus a great opportunity for learning, and it motivates the learner to learn even more. Self-Assessment Exams can be used at any stage in the learning process. For example, if the participant has not done well in a certain subject area, that test can be repeated.

answer the posttest question. As the MPP has moved to selecting mostly reviews, overviews, editorials, and lightly written data papers aimed at practicing clinicians and trainees rather than experts, the number of page views has increased. Besides the fact that it is readily available through the MPP, there is little advantage to reading text online rather than in hard copy form. Nevertheless, article text does provide another opportunity for the learner to encounter the same content they have seen in one of the other three formats.

## Drills
Case drills are interactive case presentations (Figures 5-4 and 5-8; Table 5-1) that are largely drawn from the private practice of psychopharmacology; the cases are anonymized but never fictionalized. Thus, they "ring true" to sophisticated viewers because they are real and not contrived. Each drill presents an opportunity for clinical adaptation of the same material presented in the three other formats. However, this content overlap with snippets, articles, and MOA animations is not complete; instead, it progressively increases over time as the case archive builds up.

Case drills incorporate real-world applications of psychopharmacology concepts. Clinician viewers are often only drawn to learn through the Internet when they have a complex case in clinical practice that is giving them trouble. Thus, the case drills presented in the MPP are designed as if looking over the shoulder of an experienced psychopharmacologist to see how they handle issues of treatment resistance, treatment intolerance, multiple medications, integration of psychotherapy, and comorbidities. The drills deal with complex case histories that consist of multiple prior examiners and prescribers. They follow the case over several months, with iterative trial and error treatments or combinations prescribed based on the continual monitoring of outcomes.

Case drills offer the MPP participant the opportunity to see information that is not cut-and-dried and thus to develop an eye for nuance, context, and ambiguity (Small *et al.*, 2009). The viewers are asked diagnosis or factual questions or are invited to give an opinion on treatment selection. These queries are often judgment calls without a correct answer; accordingly, the decisions of the practicing psychopharmacologist are sometimes unsuccessful, requiring reassessment and redirection. After answering the questions, the viewer sees how other viewers have answered and is given either the correct answer (if there is one) or the case author's recommendation (if the answer is a judgment call). The participant then finds out what happened next. Several clicks are necessary to move the case along, and it unfolds a bit like a detective's investigation of a mystery. These case drills are the most popular among the four formats, with MOAs a close second.

### Mechanism of action (MOA) videos

These are animated and narrated dynamic explanations of disease mechanisms or drug mechanisms in psychiatry and psychopharmacology (Figures 5-4 and 5-7; Table 5-1). They are short and to the point, and they employ colorful visual learning strategies with engaging graphics that are often based on familiar icons and graphics from the core textbooks (Wear, 2009; Stahl, 2008). Like the snippets, the animations have increased in viewership as their running times have decreased. Moreover, the number of participants who complete the MOA after opening it has increased since dividing animations into short sections that require sequential clicks to continue viewing. Each MOA may last approximately 3 to 4 minutes and may require four to six clicks to progress through the entire video. These videos are quite popular, albeit expensive and time-consuming to develop. However, with these videos, complex concepts that would take many pages to explain and an hour to understand can be understood in a matter of minutes. Furthermore, the brevity and interactivity of these videos enhance the likelihood of viewing repetition.

### Tests as assessment tools and learning events

The MPP incorporates multiple levels of testing (Figure 5-4; Table 5-2). There is a group of tests before beginning the program ("self-assessment exams") and a major test after completing the entire program (the "final examination"). The participant is advised at the beginning of the program to take 10 self-assessment examinations of 10–15 questions each in 10 subject areas within psychopharmacology and is given immediate feedback with the correct answers. Next, the clinician viewer is advised to focus on the subject matter in which he or she has the least mastery, as it is identified by the self-assessment examination. The program recommends various traditional and nontraditional self-directed learning activities that cover these subject areas; each activity includes a pretest and a posttest and offers continuing medical education (CME) credits.

The participant is then directed to the online fellowship and is asked to complete no fewer than 24 activities in 24 weeks (Figure 5-4; Table 5-1). After completing her study of specific subject matters and 24 fellowship activities, the clinician viewer is advised to take the final examination.

After passing the final examination, the participant is invited to continue the fellowship activities and examinations weekly on an ongoing basis, selecting subject areas of new interest or that arise in the field.

## Self-assessment examinations

Self-assessment can be a powerful learning tool as well as a powerful motivator for learning. Self-assessment testing is being incorporated into recertification activities of various specialty boards, including the American Board of Psychiatry and Neurology. Self-assessments help the learner identify knowledge gaps. Moreover, adults do not like answers to questions that they have not asked, and self-assessment examinations can induce the adult learner to ask questions about certain subject areas when they become aware of a knowledge deficiency. This awareness often provides the motivation needed to master new material.

## Continuing Medical Education (CME) tests

Most of the self-directed learning activities that are available online have traditional posttests that are eligible for CME credit, contingent upon a 70% passing score. The learner is presented with the correct answer to each question.

## Final examination

An individual can become designated as a "Master Psychopharmacologist" and receive a certificate by passing the final examination of 100 questions with a score of 75% or higher. The final exam is only available after completing the self-assessment exams in the 10 subject areas as well as 24 fellowship activities. The participant learns whether they have passed the exam but is not given the answers to questions. More than one version of the test exists so that participants can make repeated attempts.

## Proctor

*Proctor* is a unique element to the program that enables training directors to track the progress of their trainees. Authorized personnel can look up the transcripts of their trainees to verify completed program elements and passed tests; they can also review the results of their trainees' self-assessment examinations, including areas that need improvement. Individuals can look up their personal transcripts and monitor their personal progress (Figure 5-9).

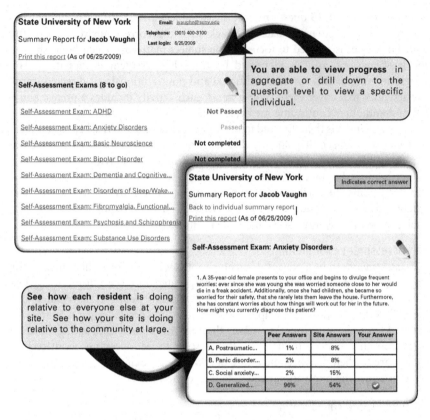

Figure 5-9. **Proctor.** Proctor is the designation for a program that allows for the tracking of an individual's progress in the MPP. It is offered to training directors who enroll their trainees. At any time, authorized personnel can look up the transcripts of their trainees to find out which elements of the program they have completed and which tests they have passed; they can also look up the results of their trainees' self-assessment examinations, including areas that need improvement. Individuals can look up their personal transcripts and monitor their personal progress. Shown here is a screen shot of a hypothetical student's progress in the program.

## Putting it all together

The MPP is adaptable to the widely varying educational needs of psychopharmacology learners. For learners who are pursuing CME credits, archives of hundreds of hours of self-directed learning activities are available, and new activities go online every week. For others who are interested in a comprehensive and organized program, the Master Psychopharmacologist certificate provides a structured learning environment that helps the learner stay on track (Figure 5-4).

Most learners want more than CME credits but don't need the structure that the certificate program offers. Instead, learners who are board certified in psychiatry in the United States are increasingly interested in maintenance of certification

(MOC). They need self-assessment examinations as well as CME and performance in practice (PIP) activities (a new component of MOC implemented by the American Board of Psychiatry and Neurology) in order to do this. PIP requires the participant to self-identify areas for improvement in their practice, take measures to improve them, and then assess whether those areas have in fact improved in their practices. Many of the fellowship activities of the MPP can be helpful in all three of these requirements. For example, case drills are a model for PIP because they assess the learner at multiple points along the case progression and give the learner feedback to gauge their responses against expert and peer opinions. The fellowship tracks their progress to see whether they perform better in subsequent similar case drills. In addition, learners who are already in practice can consult the archives of numerous educational materials and fellowship activities to immediately answer any questions that arise in their practice.

For trainees, the goal is often to become board certified – mostly in psychiatry, but also in specialties such as psychiatric nurse practitioner. Many trainees and their program directors take the self-assessment examinations (Table 5-2; Figure 5-9) and then use the MPP as a complementary resource for their own training program.

Thus, the learning principles and strategies used by the MPP are delivered in a format that is adaptable to a wide variety of learner needs and purposes without compromising educational effectiveness.

## Section 4 summary
The Master Psychopharmacology Program offers novel learning formats to address all three stages of memory formation for a wide variety of learners. The formats use adult education principles to enhance the encoding of information. The use of the Internet assists in enforcing spacing of the learning to enhance consolidation. Periodic testing repeatedly engages the recall of memory. Novel formats such as drills inject subtlety and nuance into the learning process. The program provides an overall structure to the learning but allows flexibility for individual needs (see Stahl *et al.*, 2010).

# Chapter summary

- Bolus education is not effective in producing long-term retention of knowledge because there is a rapid loss of knowledge after a single introduction to material.
- More effective learning methods can improve the initial learning but do not avoid the forgetting curve.
- The formation of long-term memory requires three stages: encoding, consolidation, and recall.
- The consolidation and recall stages of memory formation are enhanced by interval learning.
- A critical process of transferring information from the hippocampus to long-term memory storage in the cortex occurs during sleep.

- The Internet can offer great learning advantages because its flexibility is amenable to addressing all three phases of learning through expanded retrieval techniques.
- However, Internet programs may have poor compliance and must be carefully designed to avoid oversimplification of the information.
- The Master Psychopharmacology Program offers novel learning formats to address all three stages of memory formation for a wide variety of learners.
  - The formats use adult education principles to enhance the encoding of information.
  - The use of the Internet assists in enforcing spacing of the learning to enhance consolidation.
  - Periodic testing repeatedly engages the recall of memory.
  - Novel formats such as drills inject subtlety and nuance into the learning process.
  - The program provides an overall structure to the learning but allows flexibility for individual needs.

# References

CHAPTER 1

ACCME (Accreditation Council for Continuing Medical Education). *The ACCME's Essential Areas and Their Elements*. 2008.

Archer M. How to host a web conference. *Commun News*. 2004;**41**(6):16.

Baykan Z, Nacar M. Learning styles of first-year medical students attending Erciyes University in Kayseri, Turkey. *Adv Physiol Educ*. 2007;**31**(2):158–160.

Blocher D. Toward an ecology of student development. *Personnel and Guidance J*. 1974;**52**:360–365.

Brookfield SD. *Understanding and Facilitating Adult Learning*. San Francisco, CA: Jossey-Bass Press; 1986.

Chilcoat GW. Instructional behaviors for clearer presentations in the classroom. *Instructional Sci*. 1989;**18**(4):289–314.

Costa ML, van Rensburg L, Rushton N. Does teaching style matter? A randomized trial of group discussion versus lectures in orthopaedic undergraduate teaching. *Med Educ*. 2007;**41**:214–217.

Dale E. *Audio-Visual Methods in Teaching*. 3rd ed. Holt, Rinehart, and Winston; 1969.

Eaton SB, Pike MC, Short RV, *et al.*. Women's reproductive cancers in evolutionary context. *Q Rev Biol*. 1994;**69**(3):353–367.

Gagné RM. The design of instruction. In: *The Conditions of Learning*. 2nd. New York, NY: Holt, Rinehart, and Winston, Inc; 1965: 302–343.

Häkkinen P, Järvelä S. Sharing and constructing perspectives in web-based conferencing. *Comput & Educ*. 2006;**47**:433–447.

Kaleta R, Joosten T. Student response systems: a University of Wisconsin System study of clickers. *Educause Center for Applied Research Bull*. 2007;**10**:1–12.

Keller MB, Trivedi MH, Thase ME, *et al.*. The prevention of recurrent episodes of depression with venlafaxine for two years (PREVENT) study: outcomes from the 2-year and combined maintenance phases. *J Clin Psychiatry*. 2007;**68**(8):1246–1256.

Mayer R. *Multimedia Learning*. New York, NY: Cambridge University Press; 2001.

Pike, RW. *Creative Training Techniques*. Minneapolis, MN: Lakewood Books; 1989.

Pike, RW. Pike's Five Laws of Adult Learning. *Designing Training Programs*. www.bobpikegroup.com. Accessed July 15, 2008.

Price L. Lecturers' vs. students' perceptions of the accessibility of instructional materials. *Instructional Sci*. 2007;**35**(4):317–341.

Spitzer HF. Studies in retention. *J Educ Psychol*. 1939;**30**:641–656.

Stahl SM. *Stahl's Essential Psychopharmacology*. 3rd ed. New York, NY: Cambridge University Press; 2008.

Stahl SM, Davis RL. Applying the principles of adult learning to the teaching of psychopharmacology: overview and finding the focus. *CNS Spectrums*. 2009a;**14**(4):179–182.

Stahl SM, Davis RL. Applying the principles of adult learning to the teaching of psychopharmacology: storyboarding a presentation and the rule of small multiples. *CNS Spectrums*. 2009b;**14**(6):288–294.

Stahl SM, Davis RL. Applying the principles of adult learning to the teaching of psychopharmacology: audience response systems. *CNS Spectrums*. 2009c;**14**(8):412–414.

Stahl SM. *Stahl's Essential Psychopharmacology: The Prescriber's Guide*. 4th ed. New York, NY: Cambridge University Press; 2011.

Tufte E. *Envisioning Information*. Cheshire, CT: Graphics Press; 1990.

Tufte E. *The Visual Display of Quantitative Information*. 2nd ed. Cheshire, CT: Graphics Press; 1983.

Tufte E. *Visual & Statistical Thinking: Displays of Evidence for Decision Making*. Cheshire CT: Graphics Press; 1997.

CHAPTER 2

American Psychiatric Association. *Diagnostic and Statistical Manual of Mental Disorders*. 4th ed. Text rev. Arlington, VA: American Psychiatric Association; 2005.

Arbor Scientia. Data on file. 1999, 2007, 2008.

Baykan Z, Nacar M. Learning styles of first-year medical students attending Erciyes University in Kayseri, Turkey. *Adv Physiol Educ*. 2007;**31**(2):158–160.

Dacey J. The role of the society. In: *Fundamentals of Creative Thinking*. New York, NY: Lexington Books; 1989.

Drew PJ, Cule N, Gough M, *et al.*. Optimal education techniques for basic surgical trainees: lessons from education theory. *J Royal Coll Surg Edinburgh*. 1999;**44**:55–56.

Howell WS. Sending–receiving versus joint venture communication. In: *The Empathic Communicator*. Belmont, CA: Wadsworth Publishing Co; 1982;22–43.

Inscape Publishing, Inc. *DiSC Dimensions of Behavior: Personal Profile System® Handout and Overhead Masters*. Minneapolis, MN; 1996.

Knowles MS. Andragogy: an emerging technology for adult learning. In: *The Modern Practice of Adult Education: Andragogy Versus Pedagogy*. Chicago: Follet Publishing; 1970: 37–55.

Kosower E, Berman N. Comparison of pediatric resident and faculty learning styles: implications for medical education. *Am J Med Sci*. 1996;**312**:214–218.

Lorge I. *Effective Methods in Adult Education: Report of the Southern Regional Workshop for Agricultural Extension Specialists*. Raleigh, NC: North Carolina State College; 1947.

Lujan HL, DiCarlo SE. First-year medical students prefer multiple learning styles. *Adv Physiol Educ*. 2006;**30**:13–16.

Maier N. Reasoning in humans: II. The solution to a problem and its appearance in consciousness. *J Comp and Physiol Psychol*. 1931;**12**:181–194.

Mehrabian A, Diamond SG. Seating arrangement and conversation. *Sociometry*. 1971;**34**:281–289.

Middendorf J, Kalish A. The "change-up" in lectures. *Natl Teaching and Learning Forum*. 1996;**5**(2):1–5.

Myers IB, McCaulley MH, Quenk NL, Hammer AL. *MBTI Manual: A Guide to the Development and Use of the Myers-Briggs Type Indicator.* 3rd ed. Palo Alto, CA: Consulting Psychologists Press; 1998.

Riso D, Hudson R. *Personality Types: Using the Enneagram for Self-Discovery.* Boston, MA: Houghton Mifflin; 1996.

Sisco BR. Setting the climate for effective teaching and learning. In: *Creating Environments for Effective Adult Learning.* San Francisco, CA: Jossey-Bass; 1991: 41–50.

Stuart J, Rutherford RJ. Medical student concentration during lectures. *Lancet.* 1978;**2**:514–516.

Vosko RS. Where we learn shapes our learning. In: *Creating Environments for Effective Adult Learning.* San Francisco, CA: Jossey-Bass; 1991: 23–32.

## CHAPTER 3

Burgoon JK, Birk T, Pfau M. Nonverbal behaviors, persuasion, and credibility. *Hum Commun Res.* 1990;**17**:140–169.

Ekman P, Friesen WV. The repertoire of non-verbal behaviour: categories, origins, usage and codings. *Semiotics.* 1969;**1**:49–98.

Fry R, Smith GF. Effects of feedback and eye contact on performance of a digit-coding task. *J Soc Psychol.* 1975;**96**(1):145–146.

Fullwood C, Doherty-Sneddon G. Effect of gazing at the camera during a video link on recall. *Appl Ergonomics.* 2006;**37**(2):167–175.

Hall ET. Proxemics. *Curr Anthropol.* 1968;**9**(2–3):83–108.

Inscape Publishing, Inc. *DiSC Dimensions of Behavior: Personal Profile System®* Handout and Overhead Masters. Minneapolis, MN; 1996.

Mehrabian A. The double-edged message. In: *Silent Messages.* Belmont, CA: Wadsworth Publishing Company; 1971: 40–56.

Mehrabian A, Ferris SR. Inference of attitudes from nonverbal communication in two channels. *J Consult Psychol.* 1967;**31**(3):248–252.

Mehrabian A, Wiener M. Decoding of inconsistent communications. *J Pers Soc Psychol.* 1967;**6**(1):109–114.

Myers IB, McCaulley MH, Quenk NL, Hammer AL. *MBTI Manual: A Guide to the Development and Use of the Myers-Briggs Type Indicator.* 3rd ed. Palo Alto, CA: Consulting Psychologists Press; 1998.

Robinson SL, Sterling HE, Skinner CH, Robinson DH. Effects of lecture rate on students' comprehension and ratings of topic importance. *Contemp Educ Psychol.* 1997;**22**(2):260–267.

## CHAPTER 4

Arbor Scientia. Data on file (antipsychotic promotion). 2007.

Brookfield SD. *Understanding and Facilitating Adult Learning.* San Francisco, CA: Jossey-Bass Press, 1986.

Davis N. Continuing education meetings and workshops: effects on professional practice and health care outcomes (Cochrane Review). *J Continuing Education Health Professions.* 2001;**21**:187–191.

Davis D. Continuing education, guideline implementation, and the emerging transdisciplinary field of knowledge translation. *J Continuing Education Health Professions*. 2006;**26**:5–12.

Davis DA, Thomson MA, Oxman AD, Haynes RB. Evidence for the effectiveness of CME: a review of 50 randomized controlled trials. *JAMA*. 1992;**268**:1111–1117.

Davis DA, Thomson MA, Oxman AD, Haynes RB. Changing physician performance: a systematic review of the effect of continuing medical education strategies. *JAMA*. 1995;**274**:700–705.

Davis D, O'Brien MAT, Freemantle N, Wolf FM, Mazmanian P, Taylor-Vaisey A. Impact of formal continuing medical education: do conferences, workshops, rounds, and other traditional continuing education activities change physician behavior or health care outcomes? *JAMA*. 1999;**282**(9):867–874.

Fox RD, Bennett NL. Learning and change: implications for continuing medical education. *BMJ*. 1998;**316**:466–468.

Fox RD, Mazmanian PE, Putman RW. *Changing and Learning in the Lives of Physicians*. New York, NY: Praeger, 1989.

Gagné RM. *The Conditions of Learning and Theory of Instruction*. 4th ed. New York, NY: Holt, Rhinehart, and Winston, 1985.

Hodges B, Inch C, Silver I. Improving the psychiatric knowledge, skills and attitudes of primary care physicians, 1950–2000: a review. *Am J Psychiatry*. 2001;**158**:1579–1586.

Kirkpatrick D. *Evaluating Training Programs*. San Francisco, CA: Berrett-Koehler Publishers Inc; 1994.

Kirkpatrick D, Kirkpatrick J. *Evaluating Training Programs: The Four Levels*. 3rd ed. San Francisco, CA: Berrett-Koehler Publishers Inc; 2006.

Kroenke K, Taylor-Vaisey A, Dietrich AJ, Oxman TE. Interventions to improve provider diagnosis and treatment of mental disorders in primary care: a critical review of the literature. *Psychosom*. 2000;**41**:39–52.

Mazmanian PE. Reform of continuing medical education in the United States. *J Continuing Education Health Professions*. 2005;**25**:132–133.

NEI (Neuroscience Education Institute). Data on file, atypical antipsychotic polypharmacy study. 2004a.

NEI (Neuroscience Education Institute). Data on file, SSRI/SNRI and augmentation strategies. 2004b.

Oxman AD, Thomson MA, Davis DA, Haynes RB. No magic bullets: a systematic review of 102 trials of interventions to improve professional practice. *Can Med Assoc J*. 1995;**153**:1423–1431.

Phillips J. *Return on Investment in Training and Performance Improvement Programs*. 2nd ed. Boston: Butterworth-Heinemann; 2003.

Prochaska JO, Velicer WF. The transtheoretical model of health behavior change. *Am J Health Promotion*. 1997;**12**:38–48.

Relman AS. Defending professional independence: ACCME's proposed new guidelines for commercial support of CME. *JAMA*. 2003;**289**:2418–2420.

Relman AS. Separating continuing medical education from pharmaceutical marketing. *JAMA*. 2001;**285**:2009–2012.

Sharma S, Chadda RK, Rishi RK, Gulati RK, Bapna JS. Prescribing pattern and indicators for performance in a psychiatric practice. *Int J Psych Clin Pract*. 2003;**7**:231–238.

Stahl SM. Detecting and dealing with bias in psychopharmacology: bias in psychopharmacology can be easily detected and may be useful in evaluating whether to use different agents. *PsychEd Up*. 2005a;**1**:6–7.

Stahl SM. It takes two to entangle: separating medical education from pharmaceutical promotion. *PsychEd Up*. 2005b;**1**:6–7.

Stahl SM, Grady M, Santiago G, Davis RL. Optimizing outcomes in psychopharmacology continuing medical education (CME): measuring learning and attitudes that may predict knowledge translation into clinical practice. *FOCUS: J Lifelong Learning Psychiatry.* 2006; **IV**(4):487–495.

Tu K, Davis D. Can we alter physician behavior by educational methods? Lessons learned from studies of the management and follow-up of hypertension. *J Continuing Education Health Professions.* 2002;**22**(1):11–22.

Wazana A. Physicians and the pharmaceutical industry: is a gift ever just a gift? *JAMA.* 2000;**283**:373–380.

## CHAPTER 5

Bell DS, Harless CE, Higa JK, *et al.*. Knowledge retention after an online tutorial: a randomized educational experiment among resident physicians. *J Gen Intern Med.* 2008;**23**:1164–1171.

Cook DA, Thompson WG, Thomas KG, Thomas MR, Pankratz VS. Impact of self-assessment questions and learning styles in web-based learning: a randomized, controlled crossover trial. *Acad Med.* 2006;**81**:231–238.

Curran VR, Fleet L. A review of evaluation outcomes of web-based continuing medical education. *Med Educ.* 2005;**39**:561–567.

Fields RD. Making memories stick. *Sci Am.* 2005;**292**:74–81.

Glenberg AM, Lehmann TS. Spacing repetitions over 1 week. *Memory Cogn.* 1980;**8**:528–538.

Johnson BC, Kiviniemi MT. The effect of online chapter quizzes on exam performance in an undergraduate social psychology course. *Teaching Psychol.* 2009;**36**:33–37.

Karpicke JD, Roediger HL. The critical importance of retrieval for learning. *Sci.* 2008;**319**:9668.

Kerfoot BP. Interactive spaced education versus web based modules for teaching urology to medical students: a randomized controlled trial. *J Urol.* 2008;**79**:2351–2357.

Kerfoot BP. Learning benefits of online spaced education persist for 2 years. *J Urol.* 2009;**181**:2671–2673.

Kerfoot BP, Bortschi E. Online spaced education to teach urology to medical students: a multi-institutional randomized trial. *Am J Surg.* 2009;**197**:89–95.

Landauer TK, Bjork RA. Optimum rehearsal patterns and name learning. In: Gruneberg MM, Morris PE, Sykes RN, eds. *Practical Aspects of Memory.* New York, NY: Academic Press; 1978: 625–632.

Lee JLC. Reconsolidation: maintaining memory relevance. *TINS.* 2009;**32**:413–420.

Maquet P. The role of sleep in learning and memory. *Sci.* 2001;1048–1052.

Marshall L, Born J. The contribution of sleep to hippocampus dependent memory consolidation. *Trends Cogn Sci.* 2007;**11**:442–450.

McKenna SP, Glendon AI. Occupational first aid training: decay in cardiopulmonary resuscitation (CPR) skills. *J Occup Psychol.* 1985;**58**:109–117.

O'Neill J, Pleydell-Bouverie B, Dupret D, Csicscari J. Play it again: reactivation of waking experience and memory. *TINS.* 2010;**33**:220–229.

Pashler H, Horher D, Cepeda NJ, Carpenter SK. Enhancing learning and retarding forgetting: choices and consequences. *Psychonomic Bull Rev.* 2007;**14**:187–193.

Roediger JL, Karpicke JD. Test enhanced learning, taking memory tests improves long term retention. *Psychol Sci.* 2005;**17**:249–255.

Sisti HM, Glass AL, Shors RJ. Neurogenesis and the spacing effect: learning over time enhances memory and the survival of new neurons. *Learning & Memory.* 2007;**14**:368–375.

Small GW, Moody TD, Siddarth P, Bookheimer SY. Your brain on Google: patterns of cerebral activation during internet searching. *Am J Geriatr Psychiatry*. 2009;**17**:116–126.

Son LK. Metacognitive control and the spacing effect. *J Exp Psychol*. 2010;**36**:255–262.

Squire LR, Bloom FE, McConnell SK, Roberts JL, Spitzer NC, Zigmond MJ. *Fundamental Neuroscience*. 2nd ed. San Diego, CA: Academic Press; 2003.

Stahl SM. *Stahl's Essential Psychopharmacology*. 3rd ed. New York, NY: Cambridge University Press; 2008.

Stahl SM. *Stahl's Essential Psychopharmacology: The Prescribers Guide*. 4th ed. New York, NY: Cambridge University Press; 2011.

Stahl SM. Methylated spirits: epigenetic hypotheses of psychiatric disorders. *CNS Spectr*. 2010;**15**:79–89.

Stahl SM, Davis RL, Kim DH, Lowe Gellings N, Carlson RE Jr, Fountain K, Grady MM. Play it again: the master psychopharmacology program as an example of interval learning in bite-sized portions. *CNS Spectrums*. 2010;**15**(8):491–504.

Storm BC, Bjork RA, Storm JC. Optimizing retrieval as a learning event: when and why expanding retrieval practice enhances long term retention. *Memory Cogn*. 2010;**38**:244–253.

Strickgold R, et al.. Sleep, learning and dreams: off-line memory processing. *Science*. 2001;**294**:1052–1057.

Sweatt JD. Experience-dependent epigenetic modifications in the central nervous system. *Biol Psychiatry*. 2009;**65**:191–197.

Toppino TC, Kasserman JE, Mracek WA. The effect of spacing repetitions on the recognition memory of young children and adults. *J Exp Child Psychol*. 1991;**51**:123–138.

Wear D. A perfect storm: the convergence of bullet points, competencies, and screen reading in medical education. *Acad Med*. 2009;**84**:1500–1504.

# Progress check answer keys

## Chapter 1

1. d
2. a
3. b
4. b
5. d
6. c
7. c
8. b
9. a

## Chapter 2

1. a
2. c
3. d
4. b
5. c
6. b
7. b
8. c
9. a
10. a
11. b
12. b
13. c
14. b

## Chapter 3

1. a
2. d

3. c
4. c
5. a
6. d
7. c
8. b
9. c

## Chapter 4

1. c
2. c
3. b
4. d
5. c
6. b
7. c
8. d

# Progress check answer sheets

## Chapter 1

1. ___
2. ___
3. ___
4. ___
5. ___
6. ___
7. ___
8. ___
9. ___

## Chapter 2

1. ___
2. ___
3. ___
4. ___
5. ___
6. ___
7. ___
8. ___
9. ___
10. ___
11. ___
12. ___
13. ___
14. ___

## Chapter 3

1. ___
2. ___

3. ____
4. ____
5. ____
6. ____
7. ____
8. ____
9. ____

## Chapter 4

1. ____
2. ____
3. ____
4. ____
5. ____
6. ____
7. ____
8. ____

# Index

Printed in the United States
By Bookmasters